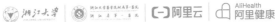

Handbook of Clinical Therapy for COVID-19

新型冠状病毒肺炎
临床救治手册

浙大一院临床实践经验

Clinical Experience from The First Affiliated Hospital
Zhejiang University School of Medicine

梁廷波　主编

U0221682

ZHEJIANG UNIVERSITY PRESS
浙江大学出版社

《新型冠状病毒肺炎临床救治手册：浙大一院临床实践经验》

编 委 会

Editorial Board

主编寄语

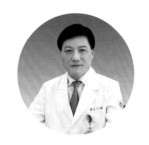

　　面对全新的未知病毒，共享与合作是最好的药方。

　　这本手册的出版，是对医务人员在过去两个多月的勇气与智慧的最好的纪念方式之一。

　　感谢所有参与编写的医务人员在救治病患的同时，把宝贵的经验汇编成册，并为全球医疗同行提供借鉴。

　　感谢来自国内医疗同行的帮助，你们所提供的经验对我们来说既是启发也是激励。

　　感谢马云公益基金会发起该项目，感谢阿里健康的技术支持，使得本手册能够为那些正与COVID-19疫情搏斗的人们提供帮助。

　　由于时间仓促，书中难免会存在一些瑕疵和不足，欢迎读者朋友批评、指正。

浙江大学医学院附属第一医院　教授

Editor's Note

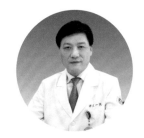

Faced with an unknown novel virus, the best remedy for us is sharing and collaboration.

The publication of this Handbook is one of the best ways to mark the courage and wisdom our healthcare workers have demonstrated over the past two months.

I would like to thank all those who have contributed to this Handbook for sharing the invaluable experience with healthcare colleagues around the world while being occupied with saving the lives of patients with COVID-19.

I would like to thank healthcare colleagues in China for giving support and sharing their experience, which not only inspires but also motivates us.

I would like to thank Jack Ma Foundation for initiating this program, and thank AliHealth for the technical support, making it possible for this Handbook to be helpful for those who are fighting the pandemic.

Due to the limited time, there might be some errors and defects. Your feedback and advice are highly welcomed!

Prof. Tingbo Liang

The First Affiliated Hospital, Zhejiang University School of Medicine

Tingbo Liang

前　言

　　这是一场前所未有的战争，全球人类面对着同一个敌人——新型冠状病毒（SARS-CoV-2）。医院是第一战场，而医务人员就是我们的战士。

　　要确保打赢这场战争，首先要确保我们的医务人员能够得到足够的资源保障，包括技术和经验的输入。再者，也要确保我们能让医院成为消灭病毒的战场，而不能被病毒击垮。

　　因此，马云公益基金会和阿里巴巴公益基金会特别邀请了一批刚刚从抗疫战场归来的优秀医务人员，在浙江大学医学院附属第一医院（简称浙大一院）的组织下，迅速总结和梳理了新型冠状病毒肺炎［简称新冠肺炎，即 2019 冠状病毒病（Coronavirus Disease 2019，COVID-19）］的临床诊治经验，并编写成册，希望可以为正处于抗疫一线以及即将加入抗疫战斗的全球各国医务人员提供一些建议和参考。

　　要特别感谢浙大一院的医务人员，他们在冒着巨大风险救治新冠肺炎患者的同时，夜以继日执笔写下了这些宝贵的救治经验。

　　在过去的 50 多天里，浙大一院收治了 105 名确诊患者，其中重症和危重症患者 78 人。医务人员在巨大的压力和风险下，创造了三个"零"的奇迹——医务人员零感染、感染患者零漏诊和危重症患者零死亡。这是奇迹，更是财富。

　　面对这种全新的疾病，中国作为最早遭遇疫病的国家，一切隔离、诊疗、防护和康复都是从零开始的。但是，我们希望这本手册的问世至少可以为其他国家的医生和护士走上这个特殊的战场提供借鉴，而不必从零开始。

这次的 COVID-19 大流行是全球化时代人类共同面临的一次挑战。此时此刻，只有不分你我，分享资源、经验和教训，才是我们赢得胜利的唯一机会，因为流行病最终的药方不是隔离而是合作。

这场战争还未结束，我们仍需努力！

Preface

During such an unprecedented global war, mankind is facing the same enemy, SARS-CoV-2. The first battlefield is the hospital, while our soldiers are the medical staff.

To ensure that this war can be won, we must first make sure that sufficient resources are guaranteed for our medical staff, including technologies and shared experience. Also, we need to make sure that the hospital is the battleground where we eliminate the virus, not where the virus defeats us.

Therefore, Jack Ma Foundation and Alibaba Foundation have convened a group of medical experts who have just returned from the frontlines of fighting the pandemic. Organized by The First Affiliated Hospital, Zhejiang University School of Medicine (FAHZU), they have quickly finished writing this Handbook on clinical diagnosis and treatment of Coronavirus Disease 2019 (COVID-19), which is supposed to be referred to by medical staff around the world who have been fighting the pandemic as well as those who are about to join.

I wish to express my gratitude to the medical staff from FAHZU. While taking huge risks in treating patients with COVID-19, they recorded their daily experience which is reflected in this Handbook.

In the past over 50 days, 105 confirmed patients with

COVID-19 have been admitted to FAHZU, including 78 severe and critically ill ones. Faced with great pressure and risks, medical staff have created three miracles: no staff was infected, and there was no missed diagnosis or patient death. This is not only a miracle, but also our wealth.

As China was the first country to be swept through by such a pandemic caused by the novel virus, SARS-CoV-2, isolation, diagnosis, treatment, protective measures, and rehabilitation have all started from scratch. We do hope that this Handbook can be a reference for doctors and nurses in other countries so that they don't have to start from the very beginning.

This pandemic is a common challenge faced by mankind in the age of globalization. At this moment, sharing resources, experience and lessons gained from the pandemic, regardless of who you are, is the only opportunity for us to defeat the virus, for the real remedy for the pandemic is not isolation, but cooperation.

This war is not over yet, but we still have to keep on fighting.

目 录

Contents

Part Three   Nursing

Appendix

References

Overview of FAHZU

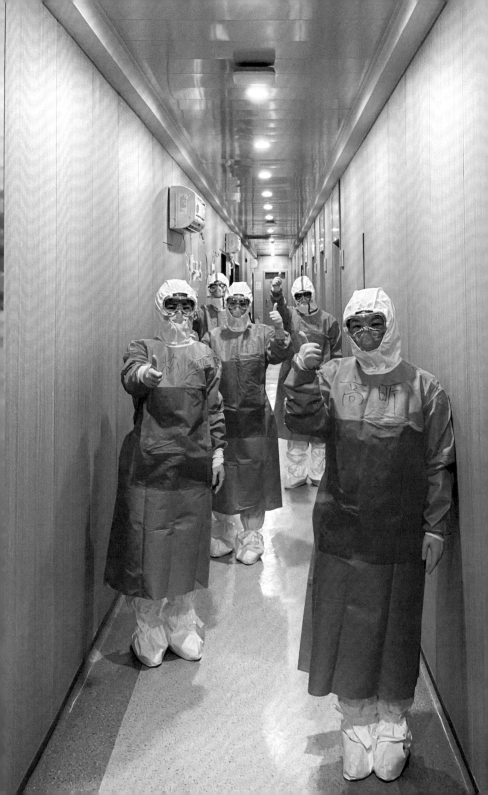

第一部分

防控管理

PART

1

一、隔离区域管理

（一）发热门诊

▶ 1. 布局设置

（1）医疗机构应设置相对独立的发热门诊，医院入口处有发热门诊专用的单向通道且有明显的标志。

（2）人员流向按照"三区两通道"原则执行。发热门诊设有污染区、潜在污染区、清洁区，且分区明确。污染区与潜在污染区之间设置两个缓冲区。

（3）设置独立的污物通道；设置可视传递间，从办公区（潜在污染区）向隔离病房（污染区）单向传递物品。

（4）制定医务人员穿脱防护用品的流程，按区域步骤制作流程图，配置穿衣镜；医务人员严格遵守行走路线。

（5）配备感染防控技术人员，督导医务人员穿脱防护用品，防止发生污染。

（6）污染区内所有物品未经消毒处理，不得带离污染区域。

▶ 2. 分区设置

（1）设置独立的检查室、检验室、留观室、抢救室、药房、收费处等。

（2）设置预检分诊处，做好患者的初步筛查工作。

（3）对诊疗区域进行分区。若患者有流行病学接触史且伴有发热及（或）呼吸道症状，则被分入疑似诊疗区域；若发热患者无明确的流行病学接触史，则被分入普通发热诊疗区域。

▶ 3. 患者管理

（1）在发热门诊，患者必须正确佩戴医用外科口罩。

（2）仅允许患者本人进入候诊区，以减少人员聚集。

（3）尽量缩短发热门诊患者等候的时间，避免发生交叉感染。

（4）做好患者及其家属的宣教工作，及早识别症状并采取基本预防措施。

▶ 4. 筛查、收治及排除

（1）所有医务人员应掌握 COVID-19 的流行病学特点与临床特征，按照诊疗规范标准（见表 1-1）对患者进行筛查。

（2）对符合疑似筛查标准的患者进行核酸检测。

（3）对不符合疑似筛查标准的，如无明确的流行病学史，但症状尤其影像学检查不能排除者，建议经专家会诊后予以综合判断。

（4）首次核酸检测结果为阴性的，应间隔 24 小时复测。2 次核酸检测阴性且临床表现可排除的，予以出院。对临床表现不可排除的，继续间隔 24 小时持续复测，直至排除或确诊。

（5）应将确诊病例定点集中收治，并评估病情的严重程度（由普通隔离病房收治或由重症监护隔离病房收治）。

表1-1 COVID-19疑似病例筛查标准

流行病学史	①发病前14天内，有病例高发国家或地区的旅行史或居住史。 ②发病前14天内，有与新型冠状病毒感染者（核酸检测阳性者）接触史。 ③发病前14天内，曾接触过来自病例高发国家或地区的有发热或呼吸道症状的患者。 ④聚集性发病［2周内在小范围内，如家庭、办公室、学校班级等场所，出现2例及以上发热和（或）呼吸道症状的病例］	符合任意1条流行病学史，且符合任意2条临床表现	无流行病学史，且符合3条临床表现	无流行病学史，符合1～2条临床表现，但影像学检查不能排除
临床表现	①发热和（或）呼吸道症状。 ② 具有以下肺炎影像学特征：早期呈现多发小斑片影及间质改变，以肺外带明显；进而发展为双肺多发磨玻璃影、浸润影，严重者可出现肺实变，少见胸腔积液。 ③ 发病早期，白细胞总数正常或降低，淋巴细胞计数正常或减少			
是否为疑似		**是**	**是**	**专家会诊**

（二）隔离病区

▶ 1. 适用范围

隔离病区包括隔离留观病区、普通隔离病房、重症监护隔离病房。建筑布局和工作流程应符合《医院隔离技术规范》等的有关要求。设置负压病区的医疗机构应按相关要求实施规范管理。严格限制人员出入。

▶ 2. 布局设置

参照发热门诊。

▶ 3. 病室要求

（1）要求分病区安置疑似患者和确诊患者。

（2）疑似患者单人单间，病室内配备独立卫生间等生活设施，确保患者的活动范围固定于隔离病室内。

（3）确诊患者可同病室安置，床间距≥1.2m，病室内配备独立卫生间等生活设施，确保患者活动范围固定于隔离病室内。

▶ 4. 患者管理

（1）谢绝家属探视和陪护，患者可携带电子通信设备与外界保持联系。

（2）开展就诊患者教育，使其了解 COVID-19 的防护知识，指导其佩戴医用外科口罩、正确洗手、掌握咳嗽礼仪、实施医学观察和居家隔离等。

二、工作人员管理

（一）工作管理

（1）工作人员在进入隔离区域前，必须接受关于个人防护用品穿脱的培训，经考核合格后方可进入隔离区域。

（2）对工作人员实行小组制模式。组内人员分时段进入隔离区域（污染区）。建议每次在隔离区域的时间一般不超过 4 小时。

（3）集中安排治疗、检查、消毒等工作，降低工作人员进出隔离病房的频率。

（4）下班前应进行个人卫生处置，并做好对呼吸道和黏膜的防护。

（二）健康管理

（1）对于隔离区域一线工作人员（医护、医技、后勤），统一安排隔离住宿，不得自行外出。

（2）提供营养膳食，增强医务人员的免疫力。

（3）为所有上岗员工建立健康档案，对所有一线工作人员进行健康监测，包括体温和呼吸系统症状等；联合专家协助解决各种心理、生理问题。

（4）如出现发热等症状，应立即进行单独隔离，并进行新冠病毒核酸检测排查。

（5）结束隔离区域工作的人员，应接受新冠病毒核酸检测，经检测阴性后定点集中隔离 14 天，方可解除医学观察。

三、COVID-19 相关个人防护管理

COVID-19 相关个人防护用品见表 1-2。

表 1-2　COVID-19 相关个人防护用品

防护等级	防护用品	适用范围
一级防护	· 一次性工作帽； · 一次性医用外科口罩； · 工作服； · （必要时穿戴）一次性乳胶手套和（或）一次性隔离衣	· 预检分诊、普通门诊
二级防护	· 一次性工作帽； · 医用防护口罩（N95）； · 工作服； · 一次性医用防护服； · 一次性乳胶手套； · 护目镜	· 发热门诊； · 隔离病区（含重症监护病区）； · 疑似/确诊患者非呼吸道标本检验； · 疑似/确诊患者影像学检查； · 疑似/确诊患者手术器械的清洗
三级防护	· 一次性工作帽； · 医用防护口罩（N95）； · 工作服； · 一次性医用防护服； · 一次性乳胶手套； · 全面型呼吸防护器或正压头套	· 为疑似/确诊患者进行可能发生呼吸道分泌物、体液、血液喷射或飞溅的工作时（如气管插管、气管切开、纤维支气管镜检查、胃肠镜检查等）； · 为确诊/疑似患者实施手术、尸检时； · 新冠病毒核酸检测

备注：1. 所有医疗场所的工作人员均须佩戴医用外科口罩。

2. 急诊、感染科门诊、呼吸科门诊、口腔科、普通内镜检查（如胃肠镜、纤维支气管镜、喉镜等）工作人员在一级防护的基础上，将医用外科口罩升级为医用防护口罩（N95）。

3. 在采集疑似/确诊患者的呼吸道标本时，需在二级防护的基础上戴防护面屏。

四、COVID-19 疫情期间院感流程

（一）COVID-19 相关个人防护用品穿脱流程

个人防护用品穿戴流程（见图 1-1）：更换专用工作服、工作鞋→执行手卫生→戴一次性帽子→戴医用防护口罩（N95）→戴里层一次性丁腈手套 / 乳胶手套→戴护目镜，穿防护服（备注：对于无脚套防护服，要加穿防水靴套），穿一次性隔离衣（根据需要），戴面屏 / 正压呼吸头罩（根据需要）→戴外层一次性乳胶手套。

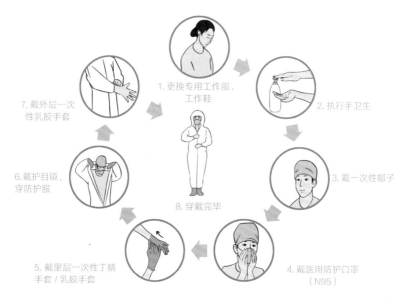

图 1-1　个人防护用品穿戴流程

个人防护用品脱卸流程（见图 1-2）：手卫生，去除外表面肉眼可见的体液、血液污染物→手卫生，更换外层手套→摘去正压呼吸头罩或自吸过滤式全面罩 / 面罩（根据需要）→手卫生→脱一次性隔离衣，连外层手套（根据需要）→手卫生，戴外层手套→进入缓冲区①→手卫生，脱防护服，连外层手套（里面反转在外，往下卷）（备注：如有防水靴套，一并脱去）→手卫生→进入缓冲区②→手卫生，摘除护目镜→手卫生，摘口罩→手卫生，摘帽子→手卫生，脱里层一次性乳胶手套→手卫生，离开缓冲区②→手卫生，沐浴更衣，进入清洁区。

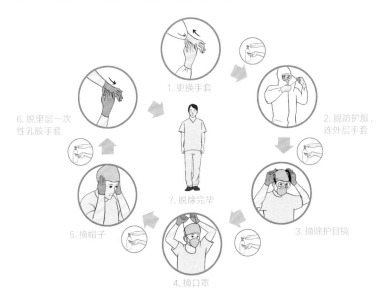

图 1-2　个人防护用品脱卸流程

（二）隔离病区环境消毒流程

▶ 1. 地面、墙壁的消毒

（1）当有肉眼可见的污染物时，应先完全清除污染物（按血液、体液等溢出进行处理）。

（2）用 1000mg/L 的含氯消毒液拖地、喷洒或擦拭消毒。

（3）消毒作用时间不少于 30 分钟。

（4）每日消毒 3 次；有污染时，随时消毒。

▶ 2. 物体表面的消毒

（1）当有肉眼可见的污染物时，应先完全清除污染物（按血液、体液等溢出进行处理）。

（2）用 1000mg/L 的含氯消毒液或含氯消毒湿巾擦拭，作用 30 分钟后用清水擦拭干净。每日消毒 3 次；有污染时，随时消毒。

（3）应按从洁到污的顺序擦拭消毒。先擦拭接触较少的物体表面，再擦拭经常接触的物体表面（擦拭完一个物体表面更换一块湿巾）。

▶ 3. 空气消毒

（1）等离子空气消毒机可以在有人的环境下使用，持续进行空气消毒。

（2）若无等离子空气消毒机，也可以使用紫外线灯进行空气消毒，照射时间 1 小时，每日 3 次。

▶ 4. 排泄物及污水处置

（1）在进入市政排水管网前须进行消毒处理，定时投加含氯消毒液（初次投加，有效氯要在 40mg/L 以上），并确保消毒 1.5 小时。

（2）消毒后的污水应当符合医疗机构水污染物排放标准，总余氯量达 10mg/L。

（三）COVID-19 患者血液、体液、呕吐物等溢出处理流程

▶ **1. 少量（量 <10mL）血液、体液溢出**

（1）方案一：用含氯消毒湿巾（含有效氯 5000mg/L）覆盖作用后去除污染物，再用含氯消毒湿巾（含有效氯 5000mg/L）擦拭 2 遍。

（2）方案二：用一次性吸水材料（如纱布、抹布等）蘸取 5000mg/L 的含氯消毒液，小心移除，并擦拭 2 遍。

▶ **2. 大量（量 >10mL）血液、体液溢出**

（1）放置隔离标志。

（2）采用方案一或方案二执行操作。①方案一：用清洁吸附巾（含过氧乙酸，每张可吸附 1L）吸附溢出液体，作用 30 分钟，去除污染物后进行清洁。②方案二：使用含吸水成分的消毒粉或漂白粉完全覆盖，或用一次性吸水材料完全覆盖后将足量的 10000mg/L 的含氯消毒液浇在吸水材料上（或采用能达到高水平消毒的消毒干巾），作用 30 分钟以上，小心清除干净。

（3）对于患者溢出的排泄物、分泌物、呕吐物等，用专门容器收集，再用 20000mg/L 的含氯消毒液按污染物、消毒剂比例 1：2 浸泡消毒 2 小时。

（4）在清除污染物后，对污染的环境物体表面进行消毒。

（5）盛放污染物的容器可用 5000mg/L 的含氯消毒液浸泡消毒 30 分钟，然后清洗干净。

（6）清理的污染物按医疗废物集中处置。

（7）使用后的物品均放入双层医疗废物垃圾袋中，按医疗废物处理。

（四）COVID-19 相关可复用医疗器械消毒

▶ 1. 正压头套消毒

正压头套消毒流程见图 1-3。

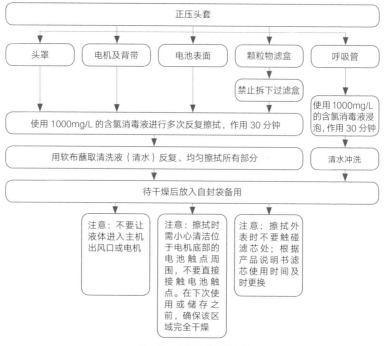

图 1-3　正压头套消毒流程

备注：以上头罩部分的消毒流程仅针对可复用头罩（一次性头罩除外）。

▶ 2. 消化内镜及支气管镜清洗、消毒处理流程

（1）将内镜及复用按钮放入含 0.23% 过氧乙酸液体的水槽中（测试消毒液浓度，确保有效使用）。

（2）连接内镜各通道灌流管路，用 50mL 注射器往管路中注入 0.23% 过氧乙酸液体，使之充分充盈，静置 5 分钟。

（3）卸除灌流管路，用一次性内镜专用清洗刷刷洗内镜各

腔道及按钮。

（4）将按钮放入含酶超声波振荡仪振荡，内镜连接各通道灌流管路，用 50mL 注射器往管路中注入 0.23% 过氧乙酸液体，持续冲洗 5 分钟，注入空气干燥 1 分钟。

（5）用 50mL 注射器往管路中注入清水，持续冲洗 3 分钟，注入空气干燥 1 分钟。

（6）进行内镜的泄露测试。

（7）放入全自动内镜洗消机，设置高水平消毒进行清洗、消毒处理。

（8）送消毒供应中心，使用环氧乙烷灭菌。

▶ 3. 其他可复用医疗器械预处理

（1）当无明显污染物时，用 1000mg/L 的含氯消毒液至少浸泡 30 分钟。

（2）当有明显的污染物时，用 5000mg/L 的含氯消毒液至少浸泡 30 分钟。

（3）干燥后，密闭打包送消毒供应中心。

（五）COVID-19 相关感染性织物消毒流程

1. 感染性织物

（1）患者使用的衣物、床单、被套、枕套。

（2）病区床帘。

（3）清洁环境所使用的地巾。

2. 收集方法

（1）第一层用一次性水溶性塑料袋包装，用配套扎带封装。

（2）第二层用塑料袋包装，采用鹅颈式封口，用扎带封装。

（3）最后装进黄色织物袋，并用扎带封口。

（4）贴上特殊感染标志并注明科室名称，送洗衣房。

3. 存储和洗涤

（1）注意与其他感染性织物（非 COVID-19 患者的）分开存放，专机洗涤。

（2）使用含氯消毒液洗涤消毒，温度 90℃，时间不少于 30 分钟。

4. 运输工具消毒

（1）运输工具专用。

（2）在运送感染性织物后一用一消毒。

（3）用 1000mg/L 的含氯消毒液擦拭，作用 30 分钟后，用清水擦拭干净。

（六）COVID-19 相关医疗废物处理流程

（1）疑似或确诊患者所有的废弃物都应被视为医疗废物。

（2）将所产生的医疗废物放入双层医疗废物袋，采用鹅颈式封口，扎带封装，喷洒 1000mg/L 的含氯消毒液。

（3）将利器置入塑料利器盒内，封口后喷洒 1000mg/L 的含氯消毒液。

（4）置入医疗废物转运箱，并在箱体外贴上特殊感染标志，密闭转运。

（5）由专人定时按指定路线回收至医疗废物暂存点，定点单独存放。

（6）由医疗废物回收机构回收处置。

（七）COVID-19 相关工作人员职业暴露处理流程

COVID-19 相关工作人员有职业暴露的风险。

（1）皮肤暴露：指被大量肉眼可见的患者体液、血液、分泌物或排泄物等污物直接污染皮肤。

（2）黏膜暴露：指被肉眼可见的患者体液、血液、分泌物或排泄物等污物直接污染黏膜（如眼睛、呼吸道黏膜）。

（3）锐器伤：指被直接接触了确诊患者体液、血液、分泌物或排泄物等污物的锐器刺伤。

（4）呼吸道直接暴露：指在未戴口罩的确诊患者 1m 范围内口罩脱落，暴露口或鼻。

COVID-19 相关工作人员职业暴露处理流程见图 1-4。

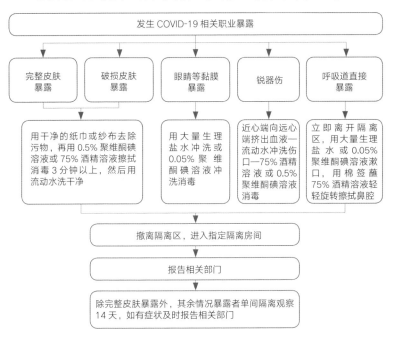

图 1-4　COVID-19 相关工作人员职业暴露处理流程

（八）COVID-19 患者相关手术感染控制流程

▶ 1. 手术室环境及人员防护要求

（1）手术安排在负压手术室。提前开启负压手术室，保持合适的温度、湿度及负压。

（2）备齐手术必需物品，尽量使用一次性的手术物品。

（3）所有进入手术间参与手术的人员（包括手术医生、麻醉医生、洗手护士、手术室巡回护士）均在缓冲间穿戴好防护用品。防护用品包括双层帽子、医用防护口罩、护目镜（根据需要）、医用防护服、靴套、乳胶手套及正压头套。

（4）手术操作人员及洗手护士在以上基础上穿戴一次性无菌手术衣、无菌手套。

（5）患者根据情况可戴一次性帽子及一次性医用外科口罩。

（6）缓冲间巡回护士在负压手术间缓冲间内负责物品传递。

（7）手术期间，关闭缓冲间及手术间门，待手术间达到负压状态方可实施手术。

（8）杜绝无关人员进入该手术间。

▶ 2. 手术后的终末消毒处理流程

（1）医疗废物：按 COVID-19 相关医疗废物处理。

（2）可复用医疗器械：按 COVID-19 相关可复用医疗器械消毒流程进行消毒处理。

（3）医用织物：按 COVID-19 相关感染性织物消毒流程进行消毒处理。

（4）物体（器械台、操作台、手术床等仪器设备）表面：①当有肉眼可见的血液、体液等污染物时，应先完全清除污染物再消毒（按血液、体液等溢出进行处理）；②当无肉眼可见的污染物时，使用 1000mg/L 的含氯消毒液擦拭并作用 30 分钟。

（5）地面、墙壁：①当有肉眼可见的血液、体液等污染物时，应先完全清除污染物再消毒（按血液、体液等溢出进行处理）；②当无肉眼可见的污染物时，使用 1000mg/L 的含氯消毒液擦拭并作用 30 分钟。

（6）室内空气：关闭层流、送风；使用紫外线灯照射消毒至少 1 小时；再开启机组自净，至少 2 小时。

（九）COVID-19 疑似 / 确诊患者尸体处理流程

（1）工作人员个人防护：穿戴工作服、一次性工作帽、一次性手套和长袖加厚橡胶手套、医用一次性防护服、医用防护口罩或动力送风过滤式呼吸器、防护面屏、工作鞋或胶靴、防水靴套、防水围裙或防水隔离衣等。

（2）尸体护理：用 3000 ~ 5000mg/L 的含氯消毒液或 0.5% 过氧乙酸棉球或纱布填塞患者口、鼻、耳、肛门、气管切开处等所有开放通道或创口。

（3）尸体包裹：用浸有消毒液的双层布单包裹尸体，再装入有双层密闭防渗漏含氯消毒液的尸体包裹袋。

（4）尸体转运：由医院隔离病区工作人员经污染区至专用电梯送出病区，并派专用车辆直接送至指定地点尽快火化。

（5）终末消毒：对病室及电梯进行终末消毒。

五、数字化支撑疫情防控

（一）降低患者就诊交叉感染风险

（1）引导公众利用互联网医院功能满足慢性病就诊等非紧急的医疗需求，减少实体医院人流量，降低就诊交叉感染的风险。

（2）对于必须前往医院的患者，建议通过互联网医院精确预约就诊时段，并给予交通、停车、到达时间、防护措施、分诊信息、室内导航等的必要指导，提前在线收集患者的全部资料，提高诊疗效率，缩短患者在医院滞留的时间。

（3）引导患者充分利用数字化自助设备，减少人群接触，降低交叉感染的风险。

（二）降低医务人员工作强度和感染风险

（1）通过远程会诊、远程多学科协作诊疗（multidisciplinary team，MDT），汇聚专家智慧，对疑难病症制定最佳的治疗方案。

（2）利用移动查房和远程查房，减少医务人员不必要的暴露风险，降低工作强度，节约防护物资。

（3）通过电子健康码和提前推送的在线流行病学调查问卷，掌握患者的最新健康状况，一方面指导患者，特别是发热或疑似患者，有效分流就诊；另一方面，保证医务人员在各个业务节点均能提前识别患者的健康状况，有效降低感染风险。

（4）利用发热门诊患者专科电子病历和 COVID-19 的 CT 影像人工智能（artificial intelligence，AI）系统，降低工作强度，快速识别疑似患者，减少漏诊。

（三）快速响应抗疫紧急需求

（1）基于云医院系统弹性扩展业务所需的数字化基础资源，即时部署疫情应急响应所需的信息系统，例如新设立的发热门诊、发热留观室和隔离病房等抗疫专设部门所需的数字化系统。

（2）利用互联网架构的医院信息系统，一方面实现医务人员在线培训并一键部署使用系统，另一方面方便系统运维人员实时远程维护，快速发布业务所需的新功能。

【浙大一院互联网医院——互联网医疗典范】

自疫病发生以来，浙大一院互联网医院快速加入浙江省互联网医院新冠肺炎义诊通道，开设专家团队义诊，提供 24 小时免费在线答疑，为全国乃至全球的患者提供远程医疗服务，让患者足不出户就能享受到浙大一院的优质医疗服务，也减少了因就医而引起的疫病播散，降低了院内交叉感染的风险。截至 2020 年 3 月 14 日，浙大一院互联网医院共在线服务患者逾万人。

●浙江省互联网医院使用说明

①下载"支付宝"App。

②打开支付宝（国内版）便可进入【浙江省互联网医院平台】。

③选择医院（浙江大学医学院附属第一医院）。

④咨询申请，等待接诊。

⑤医生接诊后会有消息提醒，打开支付宝，点击【朋友】—【生活号】。

⑥ 点击【浙江省互联网医院平台】，进入查看详情，再进入咨询。

【构建浙大一院国际医生交流平台实践】

随着疫情的发展，为了提高国际救治水平，浙大一院联合阿里巴巴创建了"浙大一院国际医生交流平台"，通过在线实时多语言翻译、远程音视频会议等功能实现国内外医生的即时抗疫经验交流，达到全球信息资源共享。

●浙大一院国际医生交流平台使用说明

①登录 www.dingtalk.com/en 下载并安装"钉钉"。

②注册账号并登录。

③申请加入"浙大一院国际医生交流平台"。

方式一：点击【通讯录】—【加入企业／组织／团队】—输入团队号【YQDK1170】；

方式二：扫描"浙大一院"二维码。

④填写姓名、所在国家、医疗机构名称后加入。

⑤浙大一院管理员批准后，按照需求加入对应的交流群。

⑥国外用户进入交流群后，可实现"图文信息交流 AI 辅助""远程音频指导""诊疗指南文件阅读"。

第二部分

诊疗经验

PART 2

本书"诊疗经验"部分内容首次发表于《浙江大学学报（医学版）》2020, 49(2).
doi:10.3785/j.issn.1008-9292.2020.02.02；doi:10.3785/j.issn.1008-9292.2020.03.01.
〔Part of PART 2 was first published in *Journal of Zhejiang University(Medical Sciences)*2020,
49(2). doi:10.3785/j.issn.1008-9292.2020.02.02；doi:10.3785/j.issn.1008-9292.2020.03.01〕.

一、多学科协作个性化诊治

浙大一院收治的主要是重型及危重型 COVID-19 患者。该类患者病情变化快，病变常累及多器官，故需要多学科协同诊治。因此，医院整合感染科、呼吸内科、重症医学科（intensive care unit，ICU）、检验科、放射科、超声医学科、药学部、中医科、精神卫生科、呼吸治疗科、康复医学科、营养科、护理部等各专科力量组成 COVID-19 专家团队，建立完善的多学科协作诊疗（MDT）机制，每日进行研讨；隔离病区医生通过互联网视频一起参与讨论，协同诊治，为每位重型、危重型 COVID-19 患者制定科学、系统、个性化的治疗方案。

科学决策是 MDT 的核心。讨论中既要发挥各学科专家的领域优势，又需集中和聚焦诊疗中的关键问题，当出现多种意见与建议时，需要由能把控全局和经验丰富的专家进行整合，确定最终的治疗方案。

系统分析是 MDT 的关键。高龄的、存在基础疾病的患者易进展至危重症。在关注 COVID-19 疾病演化的同时，需要对患者的基础状况、合并症、并发症、每日的检验检查结果做出综合分析，研判病情趋势，提前给予干预，积极采取抗病毒、氧疗、营养支持等措施，以延缓或阻断疾病进展。

个性化诊治是 MDT 的结果。治疗方案要做到因人施策、精准施策，充分考虑不同个体、不同病程在治疗上的差异。

我们的经验是通过 MDT，有效提高对 COVID-19 患者的诊治效果。

二、病原学与炎症指标检查

（一）SARS-CoV-2 核酸检测

▶ **1. 标本采集**

为提高检测的灵敏度，选择合适的标本类型及正确的采集方法和时机是十分重要的。标本类型包括上呼吸道标本（咽拭子、鼻拭子、鼻咽抽取物）、下呼吸道标本（痰液、气道抽取物、肺泡灌洗液）、血液、粪便、尿液和结膜分泌物等。痰等下呼吸道标本的核酸检出阳性率高，应优先采集。SARS-CoV-2 在 II 型肺泡细胞（type II alveolar cell, AT2）中增殖，其释放峰值（peak of viral shedding）出现在发病后 3 ~ 5 天。因此，发病初期如核酸检测阴性，还应连续随访采样检测，核酸阳性率会明显升高。

▶ **2. 核酸检测**

核酸检测是诊断 SARS-CoV-2 感染的首选方法。核酸检测按照试剂盒说明书进行，一般过程如下：对痰标本等进行前处理，并裂解病毒提取核酸，再用实时（real-time）荧光定量聚合酶链式反应（polymerase chain reaction, PCR）技术扩增 SARS-CoV-2 的 3 个特异性基因——开放读码框架 1a/b（open reading frams 1a/b, ORF 1a/b）、核壳蛋白（nucleocapsid, N）及包膜蛋白（envelope protein, E）基因，检测扩增后的荧光强度而获得结果。核酸阳性的判断标准为 ORF 1a/b 基因阳性和（或）N 基因、E 基因阳性。

多种类型标本联合核酸检测有利于提高诊断的阳性率。在呼吸道标本核酸检测阳性的确诊患者中，30% ~ 40% 的患者可在其血液中检测到病毒核酸；50% ~ 60% 的患者可在其粪便中检测到病毒核酸；但尿液标本的核酸检出阳性率很低。呼吸道标本及粪便、血液等多种类型标本联合检测，有利于提高疑似病例的诊断灵敏度，对患者疗效进行观察，并制定合理的出院后隔离管理措施。

（二）病毒分离培养

病毒分离培养必须在获得资格的生物安全三级实验室（the biological safety level-3，BSL-3）开展。简要过程如下：留取患者痰液、粪便等新鲜标本，并接种于 Vero-E6 细胞进行病毒培养；96 小时后，观察细胞病变效应（cytopathic effect，CPE），并检测培养液病毒核酸阳性，即提示培养成功。病毒滴度测定：将病毒原液按 10 倍系列稀释后，采用微量细胞病变法测定半数组织培养物感染量（50% tissue culture infectious dose，$TCID_{50}$），或采用蚀斑试验计数蚀斑形成单位（plaque forming unit，PFU）测定病毒感染活力。

（三）血清抗体检测

人体在感染 SARS-CoV-2 后会产生特异性抗体。血清抗体测定方法有胶体金免疫层析法、酶联免疫吸附测定（enzyme-linked immunosorbent assay，ELISA）、化学发光免疫分析等。患者血清特异性免疫球蛋白 M（immunoglobulin M，IgM）阳性，或恢复期特异性 IgG 抗体滴度较急性期升高 4 倍及以上，可作为核酸检测阴性疑似患者的诊断依据。通过随访监测发现，在患者发病后 10 天可检测出 IgM，在发病后 12 天可检测出 IgG，并随着血清抗体水平的升高，病毒核酸载量逐渐下降。

（四）炎症反应指标的检测

建议开展 C 反应蛋白（C-reactive protein, CRP）、降钙素原（procalcitonin，PCT）、铁蛋白、D- 二聚体、淋巴细胞总数及亚群、白介素 -4（interleukin-4, IL-4）、IL-6、IL-10、肿瘤坏死因子 α（tumor necrosis factor-α，TNF-α）、γ 干扰素（interferon-γ，IFN-γ）等能反映机体炎症与免疫状态的检测，以助于判断临床进程，预警重型、危重型倾向，并为治疗策略的制定提供依据。

大多数 COVID-19 患者降钙素原水平正常，CRP 水平显著升高，CRP 水平迅速、大幅升高提示可能继发感染。重型患者 D- 二聚体水平显著升高，是患者预后不良的潜在危险因素。发病初期，淋巴细胞总数较低的患者一般预后较差，且重型患者外周血淋巴细胞数量呈进行性减少。重型患者 IL-6、IL-10 表达水平显著上升，对 IL-6、IL-10 水平的监测有助于评估患者重症化风险。

（五）继发细菌真菌感染的检测

重型、危重型患者易继发细菌、真菌感染，根据感染部位采集合格标本进行细菌、真菌培养。若怀疑肺部继发感染，宜采集深部痰标本、气管吸出物、肺泡灌洗液和毛刷标本等进行培养。对于高热患者，应及时进行血培养。对于留置导管的疑似脓毒症患者，应同时送检外周静脉血和导管血进行培养。对于怀疑真菌感染患者，除进行真菌培养外，还建议至少每周 2 次送检血液 G 试验和 GM 试验。

（六）实验室安全防护

应根据不同的实验操作风险程度，确定生物安全防护措施。例如，在进行呼吸道标本采集、核酸检测和病毒培养等操作时，个人防护应按照 BSL-3 级实验室防护要求进行。在进行血常规、生化、免疫检验等常规检验操作时，个人防护应按照 BSL-2 级实验室防护要求进行。标本运送应采用符合生物安全要求的专用运输罐和运输箱。对所有实验室废弃物均应严格进行高压消毒处理。

三、COVID-19 患者肺部影像学表现

肺部影像学检查在 COVID-19 诊断、疗效监测及出院评估中具有重要价值。检查方法首选肺部高分辨力 CT；对于不宜搬运的危重型患者，可选择进行床旁 X 线检查。一般于入院当日行基线肺部 CT 检查，若治疗效果不理想，则 2～3 天后可复查肺部 CT；治疗后症状稳定或好转，可于 5～7 天后复查。对于危重型患者，须每日复查床边胸片。

COVID-19 患者肺部 CT 早期多表现为分布于肺外带、胸膜下、下叶的多发性斑片状磨玻璃阴影，病灶长轴多与胸膜平行；在部分磨玻璃样病灶内可见小叶间隔增厚和小叶内间隔增厚，呈细小网格状，为"铺路石征"；少数病例可表现为单发、局部病变，或表现为沿支气管分布、伴周边磨玻璃样改变的结节 / 斑片状病灶。病情进展多发生在病程第 7～10 天，可表现为病灶范围扩大，大片肺实变，内可见支气管充气征。危重型患者可表现为实变范围进一步扩大，全肺密度增高实变，呈"白肺"征象。病情缓解后，磨玻璃样阴影可完全吸收，部分实变病灶会遗留条索样或网格样纤维化改变。对于病变累及多叶，尤其是动态观察发现病灶范围增大者，须警惕疾病加重。对于具备典型肺部 CT 表现者，即使核酸检测阴性，也应隔离并连续进行核酸检测（见图 2-1）。

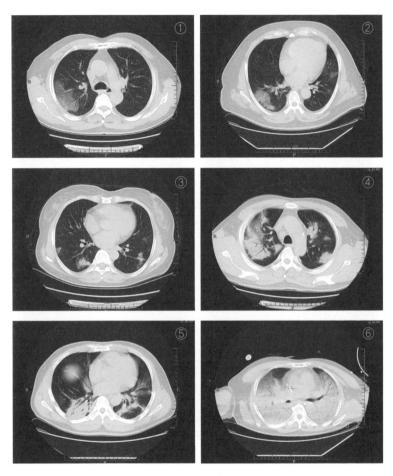

图 2-1 COVID-19 患者肺部 CT 典型表现

图①、图②为磨玻璃样渗出；图③为结节及斑片状渗出；

图④、图⑤为肺实变；图⑥为广泛实变，表现为"白肺"

四、COVID-19 患者诊治中支气管镜技术的应用

支气管镜技术在 COVID-19 患者的诊治中具有以下价值。

（1）留取深部气道标本，提升病毒核酸检出阳性率及病原体培养准确率，指导抗菌药物的合理应用。

（2）吸痰，清除血痂，解除气道梗阻。

（3）协助建立人工气道，引导气管插管或经皮气管切开。

（4）气道内给药，如滴注 IFN-α、N-乙酰半胱氨酸。

危重型患者气管镜下可见支气管黏膜广泛充血肿胀，管腔内有大量黏液样分泌物潴留，严重者可见黏稠胶冻样痰液堵塞气道（见图 2-2）。

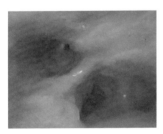
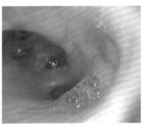
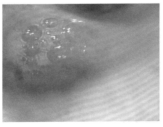

图 2-2　COVID-19 患者气管镜下表现：支气管黏膜广泛充血肿胀；管腔内见大量黏液样分泌物

五、COVID-19 诊断与临床分型

　　临床上应做到早诊断、早治疗、早隔离。动态观察肺部影像、氧合指数、细胞因子水平，以便早期发现有重型、危重型倾向的患者。SARS-CoV-2 核酸阳性是 COVID-19 确诊的"金标准"，但核酸检测存在假阴性的现象。因此，对于肺部 CT 高度疑似 COVID-19 者，即使核酸检测阴性，也可先按临床诊断病例处理，进行隔离治疗并连续进行标本联合送检。

　　COVID-19 诊断标准遵循我国新冠病毒肺炎诊疗方案，综合流行病学史（包括聚集性发病）、临床症状（发热和呼吸道症状）、肺部影像、SARS-CoV-2 核酸检测、血清特异性抗体等因素来明确诊断。

　　临床上，COVID-19 可分为以下几型。

　　（1）轻型：临床症状轻微，影像学检查未见肺炎表现。

　　（2）普通型：具有发热、呼吸道症状等，影像学检查可见肺炎表现。

　　（3）重型：成年人符合下述任何一条者即按重型进行管理。呼吸频率 ≥ 30 次 / 分；静息状态下指氧饱和度 ≤ 93%；动脉血氧分压（partial pressure of oxygen in arterial blood, PaO_2）/吸氧浓度（fraction of inspired oxygen, FiO_2）≤ 300mmHg（1mmHg ≈ 0.133kPa）；肺部影像学显示 24 ~ 48 小时内病灶明显进展 > 50%。

　　（4）危重型：符合以下情况之一者即需由 ICU 监护治疗。出现呼吸衰竭且需要机械通气；出现休克；合并其他器官功能衰竭。

　　根据氧合指数、呼吸系统顺应性等情况，我们将危重型患者

进一步分为早期、中期、晚期。

·早期：100mmHg ＜氧合指数≤ 150mmHg，呼吸系统顺应性≥ 30mL/cmH$_2$O（1cmH$_2$O ≈ 0.098kPa），未合并肺以外脏器功能衰竭，经积极抗病毒、抗细胞因子风暴、对症支持处理，恢复机会较大。

·中期：60mmHg ＜氧合指数≤ 100mmHg，15mL/cmH$_2$O ≤呼吸系统顺应性＜ 30mL/cmH$_2$O，可同时合并其他脏器功能轻中度受损。

·晚期：氧合指数≤ 60mmHg，呼吸系统顺应性＜ 15mL/cmH$_2$O，双肺弥漫性实变，需要体外膜氧合（extracorporeal membrane oxygenation，ECMO）支持，或出现其他重要脏器功能衰竭，死亡风险显著提高。

六、抗病毒治疗及时消除病原体

对 COVID-19 患者的抗病毒治疗越早越好，可以减少重型、危重型的发生。对于 COVID-19，虽然缺乏有明确临床证据的有效抗病毒药物，但根据我国新冠病毒肺炎诊疗方案，结合冠状病毒结构特征，现阶段我们可采取以下抗病毒策略。

（一）抗病毒方案

我们以洛匹那韦 / 利托那韦（2 片 po q12h）联合阿比多尔（200mg po tid）作为基础方案；使用该方案，49 例患者出现第一次病毒核酸检测阴性的平均时间为 12 天（95% 可信区间为 8 ~ 15 天），持续病毒核酸检测阴性的时间（持续 2 次以上病毒核酸检测阴性且 2 次间隔 24 小时）为 13.5 天（95% 可信区间为 9.5 ~ 17.5 天）。

若基础方案效果不佳，则可以尝试应用磷酸氯喹：18 ~ 65 岁成年人，体重 > 50kg 者，每次 500mg bid；体重 < 50kg 者，第 1、2 天每次 500mg bid，第 3 ~ 7 天每次 500mg qd。

我国新冠病毒肺炎诊疗方案推荐使用干扰素雾化吸入治疗。我们建议干扰素雾化吸入治疗在负压病房进行。因为雾化易诱发气溶胶播散，所以不建议在普通病房内开展雾化吸入治疗。

根据艾滋病患者用药经验，达芦那韦 / 考比司他的不良反应相对较轻，体外病毒抑制试验具有一定程度的抗病毒活性，对不耐受洛匹那韦 / 利托那韦的患者，在通过伦理审查后可考虑口服

达芦那韦 / 考比司他（1 片 qd）或者法匹那韦（首剂 1600mg，后续 600mg tid）代替。但不建议同时应用 3 种及以上抗病毒药物。

（二）疗　程

磷酸氯喹疗程≤ 7 天; 其他方案的疗程尚未确定, 一般为 2 周; 或在痰液病毒核酸检测结果持续 3 次以上阴性后，可考虑停用抗病毒药物。

七、抗休克及抗低氧血症维持生命体征

当 COVID-19 患者的病情从重型向危重型发展时，可出现严重低氧血症、细胞因子风暴、继发重型感染，进而发生休克，出现组织灌注障碍，甚至多器官功能衰竭，治疗上以纠正诱发因素和液体复苏为主。人工肝血液净化系统可迅速清除炎症介质，消除细胞因子风暴，阻断休克、低氧血症和呼吸窘迫的发生。

（一）酌情使用糖皮质激素

对于重型、危重型患者，早期、适量、短程糖皮质激素治疗既有利于控制细胞因子风暴，阻止病情进展，缩短病程，又可避免长期大量应用糖皮质激素导致的不良反应和并发症。

▶ 1. 适应证

使用糖皮质激素的适应证如下：①符合重型、危重型诊断者可早期使用；②高热（体温超过 39℃）持续不退；③影像学提示受累肺叶面积大（30% 以上肺叶受累），有磨玻璃样渗出；④肺部影像学表现进展迅速且受累面积明显增多（48 小时复查肺部 CT 提示进展超过 50%）；⑤ IL-6 浓度≥正常值上限的 5 倍。

▶ 2. 使用方法

根据炎症损伤程度，甲泼尼龙琥珀酸钠（甲强龙）常规起始剂量为每天 0.75 ~ 1.50mg/kg，分 1 ~ 2 次静脉注射；对于常规剂量下体温不能控制或者细胞因子仍然显著升高的重型患者，可以考虑用 40mg q12h；对于危重型患者，可以用 40 ~ 80mg q12h。在治疗期间，密切监测患者体温、血氧饱和度，每隔 2 ~ 3 天复查血常规、CRP、细胞因子、生化指标、血糖、肺部 CT 等以评估病情及疗效。如病情改善、体温恢复正常或肺部影像显示有吸收，则每 3 ~ 5 天激素减半，减至 20mg/d 后序贯口服甲泼尼龙（美卓乐），疗程根据病情确定。

▶ 3. 治疗期间的注意事项

治疗期间的注意事项如下：①治疗前完善结核菌感染 T 细胞斑点试验（T-cell spot test，T-SPOT）、乙型肝炎病毒和丙型肝炎病毒标志物等检测，避免在激素治疗过程中激活潜在感染；②根据情况应用质子泵抑制剂、钙剂预防并发症；③监测血糖水平，一旦出现血糖水平升高，及时皮下注射胰岛素控制血糖水平；④监测血钾水平，纠正低钾血症；⑤监测肝功能，及时进行护肝治疗；⑥出现多汗、自汗者，可试用中药；⑦出现兴奋、睡眠障碍者，临时给予镇静催眠药。

（二）人工肝治疗消除细胞因子风暴

人工肝系统集成血浆置换、吸附、灌流及血液 / 血浆滤过等技术，用于清除炎症介质、内毒素及中小分子有毒有害物质，补充白蛋白、凝血因子等有益物质，调节水电解质、酸碱平衡。其能阻断细胞因子风暴，纠正休克，减轻肺部炎症，改善呼吸功能。同时有助于恢复机体免疫稳态，改善体内代谢紊乱状态；有利于容量精准管理，改善肝、肾等多器官功能，以提高重型、危重型患者的救治成功率，降低病死率。

▶ 1. 适应证

人工肝治疗的适应证如下：①血炎症因子（如 IL-6 等）浓度≥正常值上限的 5 倍，或每日上升速度≥1 倍；②肺部影像学快速进展，CT 或 X 线提示肺受累百分比为每天进展 10% 或以上；

③有基础疾病而需要人工肝治疗的患者。符合①+②的患者，或符合③的患者，需要给予人工肝治疗。

▶ 2. 相对禁忌证

在抢救危重型患者中，人工肝无绝对禁忌证，但对以下患者，则须谨慎使用：①严重活动性出血或弥散性血管内凝血者；②对治疗过程中所用血制品或药品（如血浆、肝素和鱼精蛋白等）严重过敏者；③急性脑血管意外或严重颅脑损伤者；④慢性心功能不全，心功能分级为Ⅲ级及以上者；⑤低血压、休克尚未纠正的患者；⑥严重心律失常患者。

对符合适应证的患者，建议首选治疗模式为血浆置换联合血浆吸附或双重分子血浆吸附，血浆置换量建议在 2000mL 以上；如血浆来源有限，可选择血液灌流以及血液滤过等模式。具体操作方案参考《人工肝血液净化系统应用于重型、危重型新型冠状病毒肺炎治疗的专家共识》。

在我院，经过人工肝治疗的危重型患者，ICU 住院时间明显缩短，血清细胞因子 IL-2、IL-4、IL-6、TNF-α 水平显著下降，呼吸状况改善，氧饱和度提升。

（三）氧疗纠正低氧血症

COVID-19 患者呼吸功能受损以低氧血症最为突出。如何及时、有效地纠正低氧血症，缓解患者呼吸窘迫和缺氧导致的继发器官损伤及功能障碍对于改善患者预后具有重要的意义。

▶ 1. 氧　疗

（1）氧疗同时持续监测指氧饱和度：大多数患者初期氧合并不差，但部分患者氧合功能可能快速恶化。因此，建议在氧疗的同时持续进行指氧饱和度监测。

（2）氧疗时机：在不吸氧情况下指氧饱和度（SpO_2）＞93%且无明显呼吸窘迫症状时，可不给予氧疗；部分COVID-19重型患者虽然PaO_2/FiO_2＜300mmHg，但呼吸窘迫症状却不明显，也建议给予氧疗。

（3）氧疗目标：建议氧饱和度维持目标在$SpO_2$93%～96%。若合并慢性Ⅱ型呼吸衰竭，则氧饱和度目标降低至$SpO_2$88%～92%；若在日常活动下SpO_2频繁降至85%以下时，则将氧浓度提高至92%～95%，监测动脉血二氧化碳分压（partial pressure of carbon dioxide in arterial blood，$PaCO_2$）。

（4）控制性氧疗：PaO_2/FiO_2是评价氧合功能的比较准确的指标。若患者病情进展、PaO_2/FiO_2＜300mmHg，则FiO_2的稳定性、可监测性是非常重要的。推荐首选控制性氧疗。

在静息状态下，SpO_2＜93%、PaO_2/FiO_2＜300mmHg、呼吸频率＞25次/分或影像学表现进展明显时，建议给予高流量吸氧（high-flow nasal cannula oxygen therapy，HFNC），患者佩戴外科口罩。对于PaO_2/FiO_2介于200～300mmHg且患者无明显胸闷气促主诉时，HFNC的气流量应从低水平开始，逐渐达到40～60L/min。对于呼吸窘迫症状明显的患者，可直接给予60L/min的初始流量。

部分患者氧合指数较低（＜100mmHg）但一般情况较好，对于这部分患者，是否立即行气管插管，最重要的是关注原发病的进展状况，综合评估患者全身状态、代偿能力及疾病发展趋势。如果高流量（60L/min）、高浓度（＞60%）吸氧1～2小时，患者氧合指数持续降低（＜150mmHg）或呼吸窘迫症状明显加重或合并其他脏器功能不全，则应尽早行气管插管。

对于高龄（年龄 > 60 岁）、合并症多或 PaO_2/FiO_2 < 200mmHg 的患者，建议收住 ICU 治疗。

▶ **2. 机械通气**

（1）无创通气（noninvasive ventilation, NIV）：部分 COVID-19 重症患者可快速进展至急性呼吸窘迫综合征（acute respiratory distress syndrome，ARDS），而过高的通气驱动和无创通气可能加重肺损伤。无创通气导致的胃肠胀气和患者不耐受可能引起吸入性肺炎。我们不推荐对 HFNC 治疗失败的患者常规进行无创通气。若患者合并急性左心衰竭或慢性阻塞性肺病或免疫抑制，则可短期进行无创通气（时间不超过 2 小时）并密切监测，若患者有窘迫症状或 PaO_2/FiO_2 改善不明显，则应尽早行气管插管。

建议无创通气时使用双回路的呼吸机。在使用单管路无创呼吸机时，在面罩和呼出阀之间加装病毒过滤器。选择合适型号的面罩，以降低漏气导致的病毒播散风险。

（2）有创机械通气（invasive mechanical ventilation，IMV）：

1）COVID-19 危重型患者有创机械通气的原则：在保障患者基本通气和氧合需求的同时，如何降低机械通气相关性肺损伤在 COVID-19 患者治疗过程中是至关重要的。

· 严格限定潮气量在 4 ~ 8mL/kg 理想体重。通常情况下，肺顺应性越低，预设的潮气量也应越小。

· 将平台压控制在 30cmH_2O 以下，驱动压控制在 15cmH_2O 以下。

· 根据 ARDSnet 规范设定呼气末正压通气（positive end-expiratory pressure ventilation，PEEP）值。

· 通气频率为 18 ~ 25 次 / 分，允许适度的高碳酸血症。

· 当潮气量过大、平台压和驱动压过高时，加强镇静镇痛甚至给予肌肉松弛药。

2）肺复张：可能改善 ARDS 患者肺病变的不均一性，但 ARDS 患者同时存在严重的呼吸、循环并发症。我们不推荐常规应用肺复张手法；若要使用，首先应评估肺可复张性。

（3）俯卧位通气：大多数 COVID-19 危重型患者对俯卧位通气有良好的反应，其氧合和肺部力学可在短时间内得到明显改善。我们建议对 $PaO_2/FiO_2 < 150mmHg$ 或影像学表现较重的患者在无禁忌的情况下常规进行俯卧位通气，每次 16 小时以上。对于仰卧位 4 小时以上的患者，若 PaO_2/FiO_2 仍大于 150mmHg，则可暂停俯卧位通气。

对于尚未插管、无明显呼吸窘迫但氧合较差、影像学表现为明显的肺重力依赖区实变的患者，可尝试给予清醒俯卧位通气，每次持续 4 小时以上，并根据效果和耐受性进行调整，每天可以反复多次取俯卧位。

（4）预防反流误吸：常规进行胃残余量和胃肠功能评估，尽早给予适量的肠内营养。推荐留置鼻肠管进行空肠内营养，留置胃管进行持续减压；在转运前停止给予肠内营养，用 50mL 空针筒抽吸；无禁忌时取 30°半坐位等。

（5）液体管理：过多的液体输注常会显著加重 COVID-19 患者的低氧血症。在保证患者循环灌注的情况下，应严格控制液体入量，对减少肺部渗出、改善氧合有积极的作用。

（6）呼吸机相关性肺炎（ventilator-associated pneumonia, VAP）预防策略：① 选择合适型号的气管插管；② 使用带声门下吸引的气管插管（每次用 20mL 空针筒抽吸，每 2 小时一次）；③ 确保气管插管的位置深浅合适，并妥善固定，避免牵拉；④ 将气囊压力维持在 30 ～ 35cmH_2O，每 4 小时监测一次；⑤ 涉及体位变动时进行气囊压力监测、冷凝水处理（双人配合倾倒，倒入预置含氯消毒液的加盖容器中）、气囊上分泌物处理；⑥ 及时清理患者口鼻分泌物。

（7）撤机拔管时机和策略：当患者 $PaO_2/FiO_2 >$ 150mmHg 时，可积极减停镇静剂唤醒，条件允许时可尽早拔管；采用 HFNC 或 NIV 进行拔管后的序贯呼吸支持。

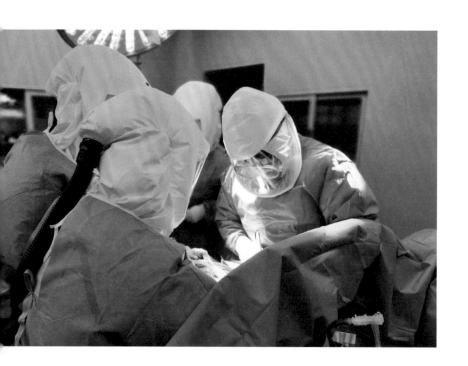

八、抗继发感染合理使用抗菌药物

COVID-19是一种病毒感染性疾病。对于轻型及普通型患者，不建议预防性应用抗菌药物。对于重型患者，需要结合具体情况谨慎决定是否预防性应用抗菌药物。对于病变范围广、气道分泌物多、原有慢性气道疾病伴下呼吸道病原体定植史、应用糖皮质激素（按泼尼松计）≥ 20mg × 7d 等情况的患者，可考虑酌情应用抗菌药物，可选药物包括喹诺酮类、第二或第三代头孢菌素、β - 内酰胺酶抑制剂复方制剂等。对于危重型患者尤其接受有创机械通气的患者，可考虑预防性应用抗菌药物，根据患者个体高危因素选择抗菌药物，包括碳青霉烯类、β - 内酰胺酶抑制剂复方制剂、利奈唑胺、万古霉素。

在治疗期间，须密切监测患者的症状、体征及血常规、CRP、降钙素原等指标，若病情发生变化，则须临床做出综合判断，在不能排除继发感染时，须第一时间留取合格的标本进行涂片、培养，及进行核酸、抗原抗体检测，以便尽早明确感染病原体。若出现下述情况，则可经验性应用抗菌药物：①咳痰增多，痰液颜色变深，尤其是出现黄脓痰；②体温升高，且不能用原发疾病加重解释；③白细胞、中性粒细胞数显著增多；④降钙素原浓度 ≥ 0.5ng/mL；⑤出现病毒感染无法解释的氧合指数恶化或循环障碍及其他提示细菌感染的病情改变。

病毒感染所造成的细胞免疫功能下降，及糖皮质激素和（或）广谱抗菌药物的应用等因素会导致部分 COVID-19 患者有继发真菌感染的风险。因此，我们需对危重型患者行呼吸道分泌物微生物监测，包括涂片、培养；对于可疑患者，及时检测血或支气管肺泡灌洗液 D- 葡聚糖（G 试验）、半乳甘露聚糖（GM 试验）。

对于以下患者，须警惕存在侵袭性念珠菌病的可能性，可考虑给予氟康唑或棘白菌素类抗真菌治疗：①应用广谱抗菌药物 7 天及以上；②接受胃肠外营养支持；③ 接受有创检查或治疗；④两个及以上部位来源的标本念珠菌培养结果呈阳性；⑤真菌 D- 葡聚糖水平明显升高。

对于以下患者，须警惕存在侵袭性肺曲霉病的可能性，可考虑给予伏立康唑、泊沙康唑或棘白菌素类治疗：①应用糖皮质激素 7 天及以上；②中性粒细胞减少或缺乏；③有慢性阻塞性肺疾病（chronic obstructive pulmonary disease，COPD）且既往气道标本曲霉培养结果呈阳性；④曲霉半乳甘露聚糖水平明显升高。

九、肠道微生态平衡营养支持

由于受到病毒直接侵犯肠道黏膜、抗病毒抗感染药物治疗等的影响，部分 COVID-19 患者会合并腹痛、腹泻等消化道症状。经检测，COVID-19 患者存在肠道微生态失衡，表现为肠道的乳酸杆菌、双歧杆菌等有益菌明显减少。肠道微生态失衡可能导致肠道细菌异位，引起继发感染，因此要重视肠道微生态调节剂和营养支持对维持微生态平衡的作用。

（一）微生态制剂干预

1. 微生态调节剂可减少细菌移位与继发感染。微生态调节剂可增加肠道优势菌，抑制肠道有害菌，减少毒素产生，减少菌群失调导致的感染。

2. 微生态调节剂可改善患者的消化道症状。对于部分出现消化道症状的患者，微生态调节剂可以通过抑制肠黏膜萎缩，使粪便中的水分减少，从而改善粪便性状和次数，减轻腹泻等症状。

3. 有条件的医院可进行肠道菌群分析。根据菌群分析结果，尽早发现肠道菌群紊乱，及早调整抗菌药物，给予益生菌制剂，减少肠道菌群移位和肠源性感染的发生。

4. 肠内营养支持是维持肠道微生态平衡的一种重要手段。在有效评估营养风险、胃肠道功能以及误吸风险的基础上，及时实施肠内营养支持。

（二）营养支持

重型和危重型 COVID-19 患者在严重应激状态下，存在较高的发生营养不良的风险。早期营养评估、胃肠道功能评估、误吸风险评估和及时给予营养支持对患者的预后很重要。

（1）首选经口进食：早期开通肠内营养，提供营养支持，滋养肠道，改善肠黏膜屏障及肠道免疫功能，维持肠道微生态。

（2）肠内营养路径：重型和危重型患者往往有急性胃肠功能损伤，表现为腹胀、腹泻甚至胃瘫。对于气管插管患者，建议留置空肠营养管，行幽门后喂养。

（3）营养液选择：对于肠道损伤患者，建议选择预消化的短肽制剂，便于肠道吸收和利用；对于肠道功能较好的患者，可以选择热量较高的整蛋白制剂；对于血糖水平高的患者，可以考虑选择适合控制血糖的营养制剂。

（4）热量供应：按 25 ~ 30kcal/kg 体重给予，目标蛋白量为 1.2 ~ 2.0g/（kg·d）。

（5）营养输注方式：营养泵匀速输注，从小剂量开始逐步加量，有条件的可以行营养液加热，减少喂养不耐受。

（6）肠外营养支持：对于有误吸高风险的老年患者和腹胀明显的患者，可考虑暂行肠外营养支持，待病情好转后再逐步过渡到自主饮食或肠内营养支持。

十、COVID-19 患者的 ECMO 支持

COVID-19 是以肺泡为主要攻击靶点的新型高传染性疾病。在重症患者，病变主要累及肺部，导致严重呼吸衰竭。体外膜氧合（extracorporeal membrane oxygenation，ECMO）治疗应用于 COVID-19 患者需要关注干预时机与方式、抗凝与出血、与机械通气的配合、清醒 ECMO 与早期康复训练、撤机标准、合并症处置等。

（一）ECMO 干预时机

▶ 1. 挽救性 ECMO

在机械通气支持的状态下，72 小时内采取保护性通气策略及俯卧位通气等措施，若发生以下情况之一，则需要考虑进行挽救性 ECMO 干预。

（1）PaO_2/FiO_2 < 80mmHg（无论 PEEP 水平如何）。

（2）Plat ≤ 30cmH_2O，$PaCO_2$ > 55mmHg。

（3）出现气胸，漏气量 > 1/3 的潮气量，持续时间 > 48 小时。

（4）循环恶化，去甲肾上腺素剂量 > 1μg/(kg·min)。

（5）进行体外心肺复苏（extracorporeal cardio-pulmonary resuscitation，ECPR）。

▶ 2. 替代性 ECMO

对于病情评估认为患者不适合长时间进行机械通气维持，无法达到预期目标的，立即采取 ECMO 进行替代治疗。若出现以下情况之一，应该考虑给予替代性 ECMO。

（1）肺顺应性减退，采取肺复张干预方法后，呼吸系统顺应性 < 10mL/cmH$_2$O。

（2）纵隔气肿或者皮下气肿持续加重，并且预期 48 小时内无法降低机械通气支持参数。

（3）PaO$_2$/FiO$_2$ < 100mmHg，采用常规方法在 72 小时内无法改善患者病情。

▶ 3. 早期清醒 ECMO

部分患者经过评估，认为其使用机械通气预期高参数的维持时间 > 7 天，且符合清醒 ECMO 的必要条件，并且患者可能从中获益的，则可以给予早期清醒 ECMO 支持。给予早期清醒 ECMO 支持的情况需要符合以下所有标准。

（1）患者意识清醒，有充分的配合度，能够理解 ECMO 运行的方式和维护要求。

（2）患者无合并神经肌肉疾病。

（3）Murry 肺部损伤评分 > 2.5 分。

（4）肺部分泌物不多，人工辅助吸引间隔时间 > 4 小时。

（5）血流动力学稳定，无须应用血管活性药物辅助。

（二）置管方式

多数 COVID-19 患者的 ECMO 维持时间 > 7 天，应尽量采取 Seldinger 方法在超声引导下进行外周置管，减少切开置管所造成的出血损伤与感染的风险，尤其对于行早期清醒 ECMO 的患者。对血管条件差、无法通过超声方法判断选择合适插管的患者，或者使用 Seldinger 方法置管失败的患者，才考虑进行切开置管。

（三）模式选择

1. 对于单纯呼吸功能损伤的患者，首选 V-V 模式，不应该为了可能发生的循环问题而首选 V-A 模式。

2. 对于合并心功能损伤的呼吸衰竭患者 $PaO_2/FiO_2 < 100mmHg$，需要采用 V-A-V 模式，总流量应该大于 6L/min，采取限流方式维持 V/A = 0.5/0.5。

3. 若 COVID-19 患者无严重呼吸衰竭，但是合并严重心血管事件导致心源性休克，则应该采用 V-A 模式 ECMO 辅助，但仍然需要给予间歇正压通气（invasive positive pressure ventilation，IPPV）支持，且避免进行清醒 ECMO 支持。

（四）流量设定与氧供目标

1. 初始流量 > 80% 的心排血量（cardiac output，CO），且自循环比例 <30%。

2. 维持过程中应保持 $SpO_2 > 90\%$，且机械通气或其他氧疗支持 $FiO_2 < 0.5$。

3. 为保证目标流量，体重 80kg 以下的患者首选 22Fr 静脉引流管，80kg 及以上的患者选择 24Fr 静脉引流管。

（五）通气目标设定

调节 ECMO 气流量，维持正常通气目标。

（1）初始气流调节，血流量：气流量 =1：1，基本目标维持 $PaCO_2 \leq 45mmHg$；对于合并 COPD 的患者，$PaCO_2$ 应该保持在 80% 的基础水平以下。

（2）应该保留患者自主呼吸，保持自主呼吸频率（spontaneous respiratory frequency）在 10 ~ 20 次 / 分，患者无呼吸困难主诉。

（3）V-A 模式气流量设定应该保证氧合器膜后血流 pH 在 7.35 ~ 7.45。

（六）抗凝与出血防范

（1）初始上机肝素应用：对于无活动性出血及无内脏出血且血小板计数 > $50×10^9$/L 的患者，肝素首剂负荷量推荐 50IU/kg。对于合并出血或血小板计数 < $50×10^9$/L 的患者，肝素首剂负荷量 25IU/kg。

（2）抗凝维持剂量目标建议：以活化凝血酶原时间（activated partial thromboplastin time，APTT）40 ~ 60 秒为目标，同时参考 D- 二聚体的水平变化趋势。

（3）无肝素运行建议：对于出现需要控制的活动性出血或者致命性出血，在无法停止 ECMO 支持的情况下，全肝素涂层环路与插管且血流量 > 3L/min，可以考虑进行无肝素运行，建议运行时间 < 24 小时，且需要准备替换的设备与耗材。

（4）关于肝素抵抗：在部分肝素使用的条件下，若出现 APTT 无法达标且发生凝血的情况，则应该监测血浆抗凝血酶 III（antithrombase III，AT III）活性；若出现 AT III 活性降低，则需要补充新鲜冰冻血浆以恢复对肝素的敏感性。

（5）关于肝素相关性血小板减少症（heparin induced thrombopenia，HIT）：若怀疑发生了 HIT，则建议采用血浆置换治疗或者阿加曲班药物替代治疗。

（七）ECMO 合并机械通气的撤离

1. 对于行 V-V ECMO 合并机械通气的患者，如符合清醒 ECMO 条件，则建议首先尝试撤除人工气道，除非已合并 ECMO 相关并发症，或者预期撤除所有机械辅助时间 < 48 小时。

2. 对于气道分泌物过多，需要频繁辅助人工吸引清除，且预计需要长时间机械通气的患者，符合 $PaO_2/FiO_2 > 150mmHg$ 的时间 > 48 小时，肺部影像学表现好转、稳定，机械通气压力相关损伤已经得到控制，可以先撤除 ECMO 辅助，不建议保留 ECMO 插管。

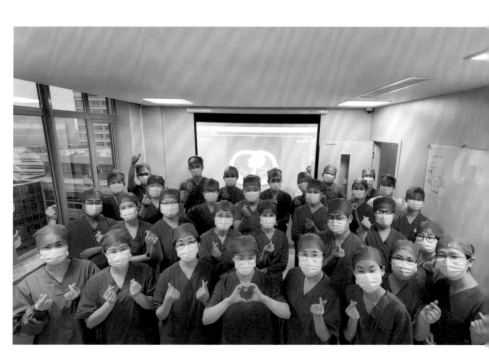

十一、COVID-19 康复者恢复期血浆治疗

自从 1891 年 Behring 及 Kitasato 报道白喉抗毒素血浆有治疗效果以来，血浆治疗已成为应对急性传染病的一项重要的病原体免疫治疗手段。新发突发传染病重症和危重症患者病情进展迅速，起病早期病原体直接损伤靶器官，进而诱导严重的免疫病理损伤，被动免疫抗体能够高效、直接中和病原体，减少靶器官损伤，进而阻断随后的免疫病理损伤。WHO 在全球多次重大疫病暴发期间亦强调，恢复期血浆治疗位于潜在疗法列表的前端，并且曾被用于应对其他疾病的暴发。自 COVID-19 疫情暴发以来，由于无特效治疗手段，初期患者的病死率较高，全社会高度关注疫情，所以避免民众发生恐慌的关键是找到能有效降低其危重症患者病死率的临床治疗手段。浙大一院作为浙江省省级定点收治医院，承担杭州地区部分患者和全省各地市危重症患者的临床救治工作，对潜在的恢复期血浆供体进行储备，同时为需接受治疗的患者及时申请输注。

（一）血浆采集

除满足常规无偿献血的健康要求，并遵循相应流程外，还应注意以下内容。

▶ 1. 采集对象

血浆采集对象包括：康复出院满 2 周（深部呼吸道样本新冠病毒核酸检测转阴时间≥14 天）；18 周岁≤患者年龄≤55 周岁；男性体重 > 50kg，女性体重 > 45kg；糖皮质激素停用时间≥1 周；

距离上一次献血的时间 > 2 周。

▶ 2. 采集方法

采集方法为单采血浆，每次 200 ~ 400mL（根据健康征询情况）。

▶ 3. 采集后检测

血浆样本在采集后，除进行一般质量检测和血液传播疾病相关检测外，还应当送检以下几项。

（1）SARS-CoV-2 病毒核酸检测。

（2）稀释 160 倍进行 SARS-CoV-2 特异性 IgG、IgM 定性试验检测，或稀释 320 倍进行总抗体定性试验检测，有条件的还应当保留 3mL 以上的血浆用于病毒中和试验。

应当注意的是，我们在比对病毒中和试验滴度及发光法 IgG 抗体定量检测的数据时发现，目前的 SARS-CoV-2 特异性 IgG 抗体检测不能很好地体现血浆实际病毒中和能力，所以建议首选病毒中和试验，或选择稀释 320 倍后的血浆总抗体水平检测。

（二）恢复期血浆临床应用

▶ 1. 适应证

（1）呼吸道样本病毒核酸检测阳性的重型、危重型 COVID-19 患者。

（2）非重型、危重型患者如存在免疫抑制情况或病毒核酸检测 Ct 值较低，且肺部病灶迅速进展的情况。

注：原则上，恢复期血浆不建议用于病程 > 3 周的 COVID-19 患者，但我们在实际临床应用中发现，给病程 > 3 周且呼吸道样本病毒核酸检测持续阳性的患者应用恢复期血浆治疗，能起到加快病毒清除，增加患者血液淋巴细胞和自然杀伤细

胞（natural killer cell，NK cell）数量，降低血乳酸水平，以及改善肾功能的作用。

▶ 2. 禁忌证

（1）既往有血浆输注过敏史及枸橼酸钠、亚甲蓝过敏史。

（2）有自身免疫性疾病病史、选择性 IgA 缺乏症的患者，应当在经临床医师评估后谨慎使用。

▶ 3. 输注方案

输注方案通常是给予 1 次输注量（输注量 ≥ 400mL），或给予多次（每次的量 ≥ 200mL）的恢复期血浆治疗。

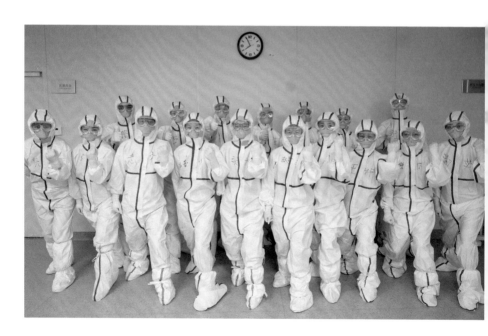

十二、中医分型治疗

（一）分型分期

COVID-19 按病程发展可分为初期、中期、重症期及恢复期。初期以寒湿郁肺和外寒内热两型为主；中期以寒热错杂为先；重症期为疫毒内闭多见；恢复期重在肺脾气虚。该病初期为寒湿证，因兼有发热，故可以寒热并用。中期寒湿热兼见，中医属寒热错杂，故寒热并用，调其升降。中医之治则"热者寒之"，治热以寒，但寒药易伤阳，导致脾胃虚寒，出现中焦寒热错杂之象，故也需寒热并用。该病以寒热错杂证常见，采用寒热并用法取得了优于其他疗法的效果。

（二）分型论治

▶ 1. 寒湿郁肺

治宜散寒化湿，芳香解表。药选麻黄 6g、杏仁 10g、薏苡仁 30g、甘草 6g、黄芩 15g、藿香 10g、芦根 30g、贯众 15g、茯苓 20g、苍术 12g、厚朴 12g。

▶ 2. 外寒内热

治宜清泄肺热，辛凉解表。药选麻黄 9g、生石膏 30g、杏仁 10g、甘草 6g、黄芩 15g、瓜蒌皮 20g、枳壳 15g、厚朴 12g、肺形草 20g、桑白皮 15g、半夏 12g、茯苓 20g、桔梗 9g。

▶ 3. 寒热错杂

治宜平调寒热，分消湿热。药选半夏 12g、黄芩 15g、黄连 6g、干姜 6g、大枣 15g、葛根 30g、木香 10g、茯苓 20g、浙贝母 15g、薏苡仁 30g、甘草 6g。

▶ 4. 疫毒内闭

治宜清热解毒，镇惊开窍。以安宫牛黄丸灌服治疗。

▶ 5. 肺脾气虚

治宜健脾益肺，补气固表。药选黄芪 30g、党参 20g、炒白术 15g、茯苓 20g、砂仁 6g、黄精 15g、半夏 10g、陈皮 6g、山药 20g、莲子 15g、大枣 15g。

以上按分型选用相应处方，每日一剂，水煎两次，早晚分服。

十三、COVID-19 患者用药管理

COVID-19 患者合并基础疾病、用药种类复杂，又往往涉及特殊人群，故临床药物治疗时应关注药物不良反应和药物之间的相互作用，避免发生药源性器官损伤，并提高救治成功率。

（一）甄别药物不良反应

相关研究显示，应用以洛匹那韦联合阿比多尔为主的抗病毒方案，肝功能异常的发生率为 51.9%。多元分析显示，抗病毒药物和合并用药数是造成患者肝功能异常的独立危险因素。因此，应加强患者药物不良反应监测，减少不必要的合并用药。抗病毒药物的主要不良反应如下。

（1）洛匹那韦 / 利托那韦和达芦那韦 / 考比司他：可引起腹泻、恶心、呕吐，肝酶水平与黄疸指数升高，血脂异常，乳酸水平增高等不良反应，停药后可恢复正常。

（2）阿比多尔：可引起肝酶水平及黄疸指数升高，在与洛匹那韦联用时，其发生率更高，停药后一般可恢复；偶可引起心率下降，需避免与美托洛尔、普萘洛尔等 β 受体拮抗剂合用，当心率低于 60 次 / 分时，建议停药。

（3）法匹拉韦：可引起血尿酸水平升高、腹泻、中性粒细胞减少、休克、暴发性肝炎、急性肾损伤等不良反应，尤见于老年或合并细胞因子风暴的患者。

（4）磷酸氯喹：可引起头晕、头痛、恶心、呕吐、腹泻、各种皮疹等；最严重的不良反应是心搏骤停，最主要的不良反应

是眼部病变，故用药前需行心电图检查。对心律失常（如传导阻滞）、视网膜疾病以及听力减退等的患者禁用本品。

（二）血药浓度监测

一旦发现血药浓度异常，应结合患者临床症状、合并用药及时调整治疗方案，实行个体化给药。需对抗病毒药物和抗菌药物进行治疗药物监测（therapeutic drug monitoring，TDM），其血药浓度范围与剂量调整原则见表 2-1。

表 2-1 COVID-19 患者常见治疗药物监测的血药浓度范围及剂量调整原则

药品名称	采血时间点	血药浓度范围	剂量调整原则
洛匹那韦 / 利托那韦	（峰）给药后 30 分钟内； （谷）给药前 30 分钟内	洛匹那韦： （谷）> 1.0 μg/mL； （峰）< 8.2 μg/mL	与疗效和毒副作用相关
亚胺培南	当日给药前 10 分钟内	1 ~ 8 μg/mL	需结合病原学检测的最小抑制浓度（minimum inhibitory concentration，MIC）解读血药浓度监测结果，进而调整用药方案
美罗培南	当日给药前 10 分钟内	1 ~ 16 μg/mL	
万古霉素	当日给药前 30 分钟内	10 ~ 20mg/L [重症抗甲氧西林金黄色葡萄球菌（methicillin resistant Staphylococcus aureus, MRSA）感染时，推荐 15 ~ 20mg/L]	谷浓度与感染治疗失败率和肾毒性相关，如浓度过高，则需降低频次或单次剂量
利奈唑胺	当日给药前 30 分钟内	2 ~ 7 μg/mL	谷浓度与骨髓抑制不良反应相关，需密切监测血细胞三系水平
伏立康唑	当日给药前 30 分钟内	1.0 ~ 5.5 μg/mL	谷浓度与疗效及肝功能受损等不良反应相关

（三）注意潜在的药物相互作用

由于抗病毒药物（如洛匹那韦/利托那韦）经肝脏 CYP3A 酶代谢，所以如有多重用药，则须仔细排查可能发生的药物相互作用，合理选择药物。有关抗病毒药物与常见基础疾病用药的相互作用见表 2-2。

表 2-2　抗病毒药物与常见基础疾病用药的相互作用

药品名称	可能发生的相互作用	联合用药禁忌
洛匹那韦/利托那韦	与经 CYP3A 酶代谢的药物（如他汀类、他克莫司等免疫抑制剂、伏立康唑）联用，可导致合用药物的血药浓度升高，导致利伐沙班 AUC 增加 153%，阿托伐他汀 AUC 增加 5.9 倍，咪达唑仑 AUC 增加 13 倍，故需注意临床症状，并进行治疗药物监测	严禁与胺碘酮（可致命性心律失常）、喹硫平（可致严重昏迷）、辛伐他汀（可致横纹肌溶解）等联合使用
达芦那韦/考比司他	与主要经 CYP3A 酶和（或）CYP2D6 酶代谢的药物联合用药时，可导致此类药物血药浓度升高；与之可能发生相互作用的药物参考洛匹那韦/利托那韦	参考洛匹那韦/利托那韦
阿比多尔	与 CYP3A4 酶及 UGT1A9 底物、抑制剂和诱导剂之间存在药物相互作用	—
法匹拉韦	①茶碱可使法匹拉韦的生物利用度上升；②可使乙酰氨基酚的生物利用度上升 1.79 倍；③与吡嗪酰胺联合使用，可使血液中的尿酸水平升高；④与瑞格列奈联合使用，可导致瑞格列奈血药浓度升高	
磷酸氯喹	—	严禁与莫西沙星、阿奇霉素、胺碘酮等可能导致 Q-T 间期延长的药物合用

注："—"：表示无相关资料；AUC：药时曲线下面积（area under the curve）；UGT1A9：尿苷二磷酸葡萄糖醛酸转移酶 1A9。

（四）特殊人群避免用药损伤

特殊人群包括妊娠期患者、肝肾功能不全患者，及接受机械通气、连续性肾脏替代治疗（continuous renal replacement therapy，CRRT）、ECMO治疗的患者等，在给药过程中应注意以下事项。

（1）对于妊娠期患者，可选用洛匹那韦/利托那韦，禁用法匹拉韦、磷酸氯喹等。

（2）对于肝功能不全患者，尽量选择原型经肾脏排泄的药物，如青霉素类、头孢菌素类等。

（3）对于肾功能不全患者（包括血液透析患者），尽量选择经肝脏代谢或肝肾双通道排泄的药物，如利奈唑胺、莫西沙星、头孢曲松等。

（4）对于CRRT持续24小时的患者，建议万古霉素的负荷剂量为1.0g，维持剂量为0.5g，每12小时一次；亚胺培南的日剂量不建议超过2.0g。

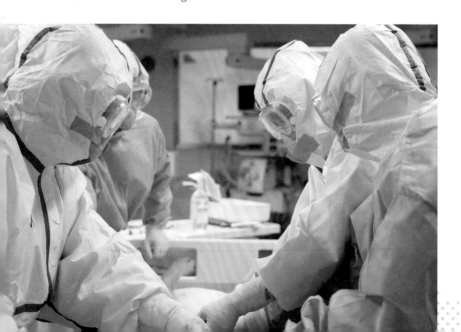

十四、COVID-19 患者心理干预

（一）COVID-19 患者的心理反应和精神症状

COVID-19 患者确诊后常常会出现懊悔自责、孤独无助、悲观抑郁、焦虑恐慌、烦躁失眠等症状，部分患者还会出现惊恐发作。在隔离病房的心理评估显示，约 48% 的 COVID-19 确诊患者在入院初期存在心理反应，且大多数为在应激状态下的情绪反应。有较高比例的危重症患者会出现谵妄；个案报道有新冠病毒所致的脑炎，患者伴有意识不清、烦躁等精神症状。

（二）建立动态心理危机评估预警机制

入院后每周及出院前动态监测 COVID-19 对患者个体心理应激、情绪、睡眠、压力等精神状态的影响程度。可采用的自评工具有心理健康自评量表（Self-Reporting Questionaire 20，SRQ-20）、抑郁症筛查量表（Patient Health Questionnaire-9，PHQ-9）、广泛性焦虑筛查量表（Generalized Anxiety Disorder 7-item scale，GAD-7）等，他评工具有汉密尔顿抑郁量表（Hamilton Depression Scale，HAMD）、汉密尔顿焦虑量表（Hamilton Anxiety Scale，HAMA）、阴性与阳性症状量表（Positive and Negative Syndrome Scale，PANSS）等。在隔离病房的特殊环境下，建议患者在医务人员的指导下通过手机进行问卷自评，医生可以采取面对面或语音连线的方式进行访谈和量表评估。在穿戴防护服的情况下，建议应用更多的肢体语言进行交流。

（三）基于评估结果进行相应的干预和处理

▶ 1. 干预和处理原则

对于轻症患者，建议采用非药物心理干预。自助式心理调适可采用呼吸放松训练、正念训练。对于中重症患者，建议采用药物联合心理干预治疗的模式。可给予新型抗抑郁药、抗焦虑药以及苯二氮䓬类药物等来改善情绪和睡眠问题。第二代抗精神病药物（如奥氮平、喹硫平）可改善患者幻觉、妄想等精神病性症状。

▶ 2. 老年患者的精神类药物选择

COVID-19 在中老年人群中高发，且中老年人群常同时患有高血压、糖尿病等躯体疾病，因此在选择精神类药物时需充分考虑药物间的相互作用以及对呼吸的影响。推荐应用西酞普兰、艾司西酞普兰等来改善抑郁、焦虑情绪；用苯二氮䓬类药物（如艾司唑仑、阿普唑仑等）可改善焦虑和睡眠质量；用奥氮平、喹硫平等可改善精神病性症状。

十五、COVID-19 患者康复治疗

COVID-19 重型、危重型患者在急性期和恢复期均表现有不同程度的功能损害，其中以呼吸功能障碍、躯体运动功能障碍、认知功能障碍尤为明显。

康复治疗在发病早期介入的目的是改善患者呼吸困难，帮助其缓解焦虑、抑郁情绪及相关症状，减少并发症的发生。康复治疗早期介入的流程是康复评估→康复治疗→再评估。

（一）康复评估

在一般临床评估的基础上，尤其注意对功能的评估，包括对呼吸、心脏、运动、日常生活能力（activity of daily living，ADL）的评估。重点关注呼吸康复评估，主要包括对胸廓活动度、膈肌活动幅度、呼吸模式和频率等的评估。

（二）康复治疗

对 COVID-19 重症、危重症患者的康复治疗方法主要包括体位管理、呼吸运动训练、主动循环技术、呼气正压训练器和物理因子治疗等。

▶ 1. 体位管理

患者合理的体位可以减少痰液对呼吸道的影响，对改善患者的通气血流灌注比值（ventilation/perfusion ratio，V/Q）尤其重要。当患者处于合理的体位时，利用重力作用可以促进肺叶或者肺段气道分泌物引流排出。对于镇静和意识障碍的患者，在生理条件

允许的情况下，可采取起立床或抬高床头（30°→45°→60°）的方法来促进气道分泌物排出。站位是静息时的最佳通气体位，可有效提高患者的通气效率，维持肺容积。在患者能耐受的情况下，尽量争取患者保持站位，并逐渐增加站位时间。

▶ 2. 呼吸运动训练

呼吸运动能使患者肺部得到充分扩张，帮助肺泡和气道中的分泌物向大气道排出，避免痰液集聚在肺底部，以便增加肺活量，增强肺功能。其中，两种主要的呼吸运动训练方法是深慢呼吸、扩胸配合肩部外展呼吸。

（1）深漫呼吸：指吸气时尽量调动膈肌主动参与，呼吸尽量深慢，避免浅快呼吸造成通气效率降低。该呼吸方式比胸式呼吸做功低，潮气量、通气灌注比优，可用于患者呼吸急促时调整呼吸。

（2）扩胸配合肩部外展呼吸：可提高肺通气效应。做深慢呼吸，吸气时扩胸，配合肩外展；呼气时含胸，肩内收。病毒性肺炎患者由于其特殊的病理性因素，所以呼吸时应尽量避免长时间闭气，以免增加呼吸功、氧耗及心脏负担。同时，注意避免动作速度过快，尽量将呼吸频率调整至 12 ~ 15 次 / 分为佳。

▶ 3. 主动循环技术

主动循环技术不仅可有效清除支气管分泌物，改善肺功能，而且不会加重低氧血症和气流阻塞。该技术有呼吸控制、胸廓扩张、呵气三个阶段，可根据患者情况选择构成方式，并进行反复循环。

▶ 4. 呼气正压训练器

COVID-19 患者肺间质结构破坏严重，在机械通气中一般采取低压力低潮，避免造成肺间质损伤，因此脱机后可采用低压呼气正压训练器来促使分泌物由低容量肺段向高容量肺段移动，降低排痰难度，减少排痰做功。通过振荡气流产生呼气正压，振动气道，达到一定的气道支撑效应，再通过高呼气流速，松动痰液，移除分泌物。

▶ 5. 物理因子治疗

物理因子治疗包括超短波、振荡器、体外膈肌起搏器、肌肉功能电刺激等。

十六、COVID-19 患者肺移植

肺移植是终末期慢性肺病的一种有效治疗手段。查阅文献发现，鲜有将肺移植用于治疗急性传染性肺部疾病的报道。浙大一院根据目前临床实践结果，总结得出以下体会，供同行参考：总体遵循探索性、抢救性、高选择、高防护的原则，在给予充分、合理、优化的内科治疗后，肺部病变仍无明显好转，严重威胁患者生命安全时，需考虑肺移植评估。

（一）移植前评估

▶ 1. 年　龄

建议肺移植患者年龄 < 70 岁；对于 70 岁及以上患者，需谨慎评估其他脏器功能及术后恢复能力。

▶ 2. 病　程

虽然病程长短与疾病严重程度无直接相关性，但对于病程短于 4 ~ 6 周者，需充分评估是否给予充分的药物、呼吸机辅助和 ECMO 支持。

▶ 3. 肺功能状态

肺部 CT、呼吸机、ECMO 参数可作为参考依据，充分评估是否存在逆转的机会。

▶ 4. 其他大脏器功能评估

多数危重症患者长期处于镇静状态，故对其意识状态进行判断是十分重要的。对有条件者，建议行头颅 CT、脑电图检查。心脏评估包括心电图、心脏超声，重点评估右心大小、肺动脉压以及左心功能情况。血清肌酐、胆红素水平都应被纳入评估范围。对合并肝功能衰竭、肾衰竭者，应待肝肾功能好转后再行评估。

▶ 5. 新冠病毒核酸检测

新冠病毒核酸检测最少连续 2 次为阴性，每次间隔 24 小时；考虑到目前复阳情况增多，建议新冠病毒核酸检测增加到连续 3 次以上阴性。理想情况是所有体液标本，包括血、痰、鼻咽、肺泡灌洗液、尿液、粪便标本病毒核酸检测均为阴性；但考虑到实际操作情况，至少痰、肺泡灌洗液标本病毒核酸检测为阴性。

▶ 6. 感染状态评估

随着住院时间的延长，部分 COVID-19 患者会合并多重耐药菌感染。应充分评估目前的感染控制情况，尤其是多重耐药菌感染控制情况，并且需要制定术后抗菌药物治疗方案，预估术后感染进展风险。

▶ 7. 肺移植术前评估流程

由重症监护室医疗团队提出→多学科讨论→完善全面检查→分析处理相对禁忌证→术前康复，为肺移植创造条件。

（二）禁忌证

参考 2014 年国际心肺移植学会（The International Society for Heart and Lung Transplantation, ISHLT）共识：肺移植受者选择（更新版）。

十七、COVID-19 患者出院标准及随访计划

（一）出院标准

1. 体温正常（耳温 < 37.5℃）至少 3 天。

2. 呼吸道症状明显好转。

3. 新冠病毒核酸检测连续 2 次以上阴性（每次间隔时间 > 24 小时），有条件的医疗机构可同时行粪便标本新冠病毒核酸检测。

4. 肺部影像学检查显示病灶较前明显好转。

5. 无其他需要住院治疗的合并症或并发症。

6. 在不吸氧情况下，SpO_2 > 93%。

7. 经医院多学科协作诊疗团队专家组讨论并认可达到出院标准。

（二）出院后用药

一般患者无须继续服用抗病毒药物，若有轻度咳嗽、胃纳不佳、舌苔偏厚等症状，则可予以对症处理；对于部分肺部病灶较多、新冠病毒核酸检测转阴时间 < 3 天的患者，可考虑出院后继续带抗病毒药物。

（三）居家隔离

出院后患者仍须居家隔离 2 周。建议提供以下居家隔离条件：①有独立的生活区，需勤通风、勤消毒；②避免与家中的婴幼儿、老年人及免疫功能低下者接触；③患者及其家属须佩戴口罩，勤

洗手；④每日测量体温 2 次（早晚各 1 次），密切关注机体变化。

（四）随 访

针对每一位出院患者，医院安排随访医生专人专管，在出院后 48 小时内进行第一次电话随访。在出院后 1 周、2 周及 1 个月的时间节点进行门诊随访，根据患者情况进行以下检查：①血液标本新冠病毒核酸检测；②肝肾功能、血常规检查；③痰液及粪便标本新冠病毒核酸检测；④肺功能评估；⑤肺部 CT 复检。在出院后 3 个月及 6 个月的时间节点进行电话随访。

（五）复阳患者的处理

浙大一院严格执行出院标准，随访中未发现已出院患者的痰液、粪便标本新冠病毒核酸检测再次阳性的情况；但已有较多报道，参照我国指南推荐的标准（间隔 24 小时连续 2 次咽拭子标本新冠病毒核酸检测阴性＋体温正常 3 天＋症状明显好转＋肺部影像显示吸收好转），发现部分患者在复诊中新冠病毒核酸检测阳性，这可能主要与标本留取、检测呈假阴性有关。针对此类患者，我们有如下建议。

（1）按 COVID-19 患者标准进行隔离。

（2）继续给予前期有效的抗病毒方案治疗。

（3）在肺部影像进一步好转，痰液、粪便标本 SARS-CoV-2 核酸检测持续阴性 3 次（每次间隔 24 小时）后出院。

（4）出院后按上文提到的居家隔离及随访要求进行观察。

第三部分

护理经验

PART
3

一、高流量吸氧（HFNC）患者护理

（一）注意事项

在应用 HFNC 前应充分宣教，必要时应用小剂量镇静药物。根据患者鼻腔直径选择合适的鼻塞导管。使用时先贴减压敷料，调节好鼻塞固定带松紧度，避免引起面部皮肤器械相关性压力损伤。根据患者病情和耐受情况，调节氧浓度、流量及温度，及时添加湿化水。

（二）病情监测

在应用 HFNC 期间，若患者出现血流动力学不稳定、辅助呼吸肌运动明显、氧合持续未改善、意识状态恶化、呼吸频率持续超过 40 次 / 分、大量气道分泌物等表现，则应及时报告医生，考虑是否需要中止 HFNC，及时行气管插管机械通气。

（三）分泌物处理

患者自行或在护士的帮助下用纸巾擦拭口水、鼻涕、痰液，并将用过的纸巾包裹后丢入预置 2500mg/L 含氯消毒液的一次性密闭容器中；或直接用口腔吸引管将口水、痰液吸入预置 2500mg/L 含氯消毒液的收集器。

二、机械通气患者护理

（一）气管插管配合

限制保证患者安全所需的最低医务人数。医务人员应佩戴正压头套。插管前，给予充分镇痛、镇静，必要时应用肌松药，同时做好血流动力学监测。在操作完成后 30 分钟内，减少室内人员走动，持续进行等离子空气净化消毒。

（二）镇痛镇静、谵妄管理

每日确定镇痛镇静目标，使用重症监护室疼痛观察工具法（Critical Care Pain Observation Tool，CPOT）每 4 小时评估一次镇痛程度，使用 Richmond 镇静程度评估表（Richmond Agitation-Sedation Scale，RASS）或脑电双频指数（bispectral index，BIS）每 2 小时评估一次镇静深度，滴定调节镇痛、镇静药物。明确会引起疼痛的操作预先给予镇痛。每班使用重症监护室意识模糊评估法（Confusion Assessment Method of the Intensive Care Unit，CAM-ICU）进行谵妄筛查，尽早识别阳性患者。落实谵妄预防集束化策略：处理疼痛，最小化镇静，沟通交流，促进睡眠，早期活动等。

（三）呼吸机相关性肺炎的预防

执行呼吸机相关性肺损伤预防集束化策略，包括：遵循手卫生制度；如无禁忌证，将床头抬高 30°～ 45°；采用一次性吸唾牙刷，每 4 ～ 6 小时进行一次口腔护理；维持气囊压

$30 \sim 35cmH_2O$，每 4 小时监测一次；经胃管管饲营养液，每 4 小时监测一次胃残留量；每天评估能否撤机；使用可冲洗的气管导管持续低负压吸引声门下分泌物，同时每 $1 \sim 2$ 小时间断使用 10mL 注射器抽吸，并根据实际囊上分泌物的量，调整抽吸频次。声门下滞留物的处置：使用 10mL 注射器抽吸囊上分泌物，然后立即抽吸适量 2500mg/L 含氯消毒液，连接针帽，放入锐器盒内。

（四）吸痰的护理

▶ 1. 吸　痰

使用密闭式吸痰管、密闭式抛弃型集痰袋，减少气溶胶及飞沫。

▶ 2. 采集痰液标本

使用密闭式吸痰管配套使用的集痰器，减少飞沫暴露。

（五）呼吸机管道冷凝水的处理

使用一次性双回路自带加热导丝的呼吸机管路、自动加水湿化罐，减少冷凝水的产生。及时倾倒冷凝水，使用预置 2500mg/L 含氯消毒液的加盖容器，双人配合将管道内的积水倒入加盖容器内后，直接放入温度可达 90℃的清洗机内进行自动清洗、消毒。

（六）俯卧位通气护理

翻身前做好充分准备，妥善固定导管，检查所有导管接口，降低脱开的风险。翻转后每 2 小时改变一次体位。

1. 由 ECMO 灌注师专人管理，每小时检查并予以记录。记录以下项目：转速、血流量，氧流量、氧浓度，控温仪是否转流、设置及实际温度；ECMO 内有无血块，管路有无打折、压迫，静脉管路有无抖动；患者尿色有无变红色或深棕色；遵医嘱监测膜前 / 膜后压力。

2. 每班检查并记录置管深度、管路固定情况，各接口是否牢固，控温仪水位线，机器电源、气源连接情况；穿刺处有无渗血、肿胀；测量双下肢腿围，观察术侧下肢有无肿胀及末梢血运情况，如足背动脉搏动、皮温、颜色等。

3. 每日监测膜后血气分析。

4. ECMO 抗凝管理的基本目标是适度抗凝，在避免凝血过度激活的前提下保证一定的凝血活性，即维持抗凝、凝血和纤溶三者之间的平衡。置管时注射负荷剂量肝素钠（25 ~ 50IU/kg），转流期间给予肝素钠维持 [7.5 ~ 20.0IU/（kg·h）]，根据APTT 结果进行调整，APTT 目标为 40 ~ 60 秒；抗凝期间尽量减少皮肤穿刺次数，各项操作动作宜轻柔，并密切观察有无出血情况。

5. 实行"超保护性肺通气"策略，最大限度地避免或减少呼吸机相关性肺损伤的发生，建议初始潮气量 < 6mL/kg，保留自主呼吸，保持自主呼吸频率在 10 ~ 20 次 / 分。

6. 密切观察患者生命体征变化，维持平均动脉压（mean arterial pressure，MAP）60 ~ 65mmHg，中心静脉压（central

venous pressure，CVP）< 8mmHg，SpO_2 > 90%，监测尿量、电解质情况。

7. 输液、输血尽量于膜后输注，避免输注脂肪乳、丙泊酚等药物。

8. 根据日常监测管理记录，每班评估 ECMO 氧合器功能。

四、人工肝护理

人工肝护理主要分为治疗期护理和治疗间歇期护理。在人工肝治疗期间，护理人员应密切观察患者病情，规范操作流程，关注重点环节，及时处理并发症，以便顺利完成人工肝治疗。

（一）治疗期护理

治疗期护理指每次人工肝治疗过程中的护理，其整体操作流程可归纳如下：操作人员自身准备→患者评估→装机→预冲→上机→参数调节→下机→记录。各环节的护理重点如下。

1. 操作人员自身准备。全面执行三级及以上防护措施。

2. 患者评估，包括患者基本情况及病情，尤其是过敏史、血糖、凝血功能、氧疗情况及镇静状态；对于清醒患者，要关注其心理状态；评估患者导管功能状态。

3. 装机和预冲。治疗管路及耗材尽量选择闭环，避免患者血液、体液暴露；按照拟定的治疗模式选择相应的仪器、管路及耗材，熟悉治疗耗材的基本性能。

4. 上机。建议起始引血速度 ≤ 35mL/min，避免速度过快导致低血压；实时监测患者生命体征。

5. 参数调节。待体外循环稳定后，根据治疗模式调节各项治疗参数及报警参数；早期足量使用抗凝剂，维持量根据各治疗压力随时调整。

6. 下机。采取液体＋重力组合回收法，回收速度 ≤ 35mL/min；下机后按新冠病毒感染防控要求处理医疗废物，并对治疗室及治疗仪器进行清洁、消毒。

7. 记录，包括记录患者生命体征、人工肝用药情况、人工肝治疗参数以及特殊情况备注等。

（二）间歇期护理

1. 观察和处理迟发型并发症，如观察有无发生过敏反应、失衡综合征等，并给予处理。

2. 人工肝置管护理。每班观察局部情况并予以记录；给予预防导管相关性血栓护理；每48小时进行一次导管专业维护。

3. 人工肝置管拔管护理。拔管前行血管超声检查；拔管后置管侧下肢制动6小时，且24小时内卧床休息，观察局部创面情况。

五、CRRT 护理

（一）治疗前准备

1. 患者准备。建立有效血管通路，一般行中心静脉置管，首选颈内静脉。如同时行 ECMO 治疗，则可将 CRRT 整合入 ECMO 系统。

2. 设备、耗材、超滤用药准备。

（二）治疗中护理

1. 血管通路的护理。对于中心静脉置管的患者，每 24 小时进行一次专业导管护理，妥善固定通路，避免发生扭曲、受压。在将 CRRT 整合入 ECMO 治疗时，需双人核对连接方法及连接的紧密性。建议 CRRT 的引出端及回输端均在氧合器后。

2. 严密监测患者神志及生命体征变化，准确计算液体出入量；严密观察体外循环凝血情况，有效处理报警，确保机器顺畅运转；每 4 小时进行一次血气分析监测，评估内环境电解质及酸碱平衡；置换液的配制应严格遵守无菌技术操作规程，现配现用，标志清晰。

（三）治疗后护理

1. 监测患者血常规、肝肾功能、凝血功能。

2. 对于持续进行治疗的机器，每 24 小时擦拭、消毒一次；耗材及废液按医院感染要求进行处置。

六、一般护理

（一）严密监测患者病情

监测患者生命体征，特别是意识、呼吸频率、血氧饱和度等的变化。观察患者咳嗽、咳痰、胸闷、呼吸困难及发绀情况，动态监测血气分析，及时发现病情变化，调整氧疗策略或实施急救。关注高呼气末正压通气、高压力支持下气道压力、潮气量和呼吸频率变化，观察有无发生气压伤。

（二）预防误吸

1. 胃潴留的监测与护理。使用营养泵持续幽门后喂养，以减少胃食管反流；有条件时采用超声评估胃动力和胃潴留情况。对于胃排空好的患者，不建议行常规评估。

2. 每 4 小时评估一次胃潴留量。若胃潴留量 < 100mL，则予以回输；若胃潴留量 > 100mL，则汇报医生后再做决定。

3. 转运期间误吸的预防。转运前，停止鼻饲，回抽胃内残余量，胃管接负压袋引流；转运时，保持床头抬高 30°。

4. 经鼻高流量吸氧治疗患者误吸的预防。每 4 小时巡查一次，避免湿化过度或湿化不足导致管路积水，并及时处理；警惕误入气道引起呛咳和误吸；保持鼻塞位置高度高于机器和管路水平，及时处理管路冷凝水。

（三）预防感染

实施导管相关性血流感染、导尿管相关尿路感染策略。

（四）预防皮肤损伤

预防皮肤压力性损伤（包括器械相关压力性损伤）、失禁性皮炎、医用黏胶相关性皮肤损伤，使用风险评估量表筛选高危患者，实施预防策略。

（五）预防血栓

在患者入院、病情发生变化时，进行静脉血栓栓塞症（venous thromboembolism，VTE）风险评估，筛查高危患者，落实预防策略。监测凝血功能及 D- 二聚体浓度变化，关注 VTE 相关临床表现。

（六）营养支持

对于体弱、呼吸急促、氧合波动明显者，应协助进食，进食期间加强氧合监测。对于不能经口进食者，早期开通肠内营养，每班评估患者肠内营养耐受情况，并根据评估结果调整肠内营养速度和量。

附　录

APPENDIX

一、COVID-19 患者医嘱范例

（一）COVID-19 轻型患者医嘱范例

▶ 1. 诊疗医嘱

给予空气隔离、血氧饱和度监测、鼻导管吸氧。

▶ 2. 检查医嘱

·2019 新型冠状病毒 RNA 测定（三位点）（痰）qd。

·2019 新型冠状病毒 RNA 测定（三位点）（粪便）qd。

·血常规、生化、尿常规、粪便常规 + OB、凝血功能 + D- 二聚体、血气分析 + 乳酸、ASO + RF + CRP + CCP、ESR、PCT、ABO + Rh 血型、甲状腺功能、心肌酶 + 血清肌钙蛋白定量、常规四项、呼吸道病毒、细胞因子、G/GM 试验、血管紧张素转换酶测定。

·肝胆胰脾超声、心脏超声、肺部 CT。

▶ 3. 药物医嘱

·阿比多尔片 200mg po tid。

·洛匹那韦 / 利托那韦片 2 片 po q12h。

·干扰素喷雾剂 1 喷 pr.nar tid。

（二）COVID-19 普通型患者医嘱范例

▶ 1. 诊疗医嘱

给予空气隔离、血氧饱和度监测、鼻导管吸氧。

▶ 2. 检查医嘱

·2019 新型冠状病毒 RNA 测定（三位点）（痰）qd。

·2019 新型冠状病毒 RNA 测定（三位点）（粪便）qd。

·血常规、生化、尿常规、粪便常规 +OB、凝血功能 + D- 二聚体、血气分析 + 乳酸、ASO + RF + CRP + CCP、ESR、PCT、ABO + Rh 血型、甲状腺功能、心肌酶 + 血清肌钙蛋白定量、常规四项、呼吸道病毒、细胞因子、G/GM 试验、血管紧张素转换酶测定。

·肝胆胰脾超声、心脏超声、肺部 CT。

▶ 3. 药物医嘱

·阿比多尔片 200mg po tid。

·洛匹那韦 / 利托那韦片 2 片 po q12h。

·干扰素喷雾剂 1 喷 pr.nar tid。

·NS 100mL+ 氨溴索 30mg ivgtt bid。

（三）COVID-19 重型患者医嘱范例

▶ 1. 诊疗医嘱

给予空气隔离、血氧饱和度监测、鼻导管吸氧。

▶ 2. 检查医嘱

·2019 新型冠状病毒 RNA 测定（三位点）（痰）qd。

·2019 新型冠状病毒 RNA 测定（三位点）（粪便）qd。

·血常规、生化、尿常规、粪便常规 + OB、凝血功能 + D- 二聚体、血气分析 + 乳酸、ASO + RF + CRP + CCP、ESR、PCT、ABO + Rh 血型、甲状腺功能、心肌酶 + 血清肌钙蛋白定量、常规四项、呼吸道病毒、免疫球蛋白 + 补体、细胞因子、G/GM 试验、血管紧张素转换酶测定。

·肝胆胰脾超声、心脏超声、肺部 CT。

▶ 3. 药物医嘱

·阿比多尔片 200mg po tid。

·洛匹那韦 / 利托那韦片 2 片 po q12h。

- 干扰素喷雾剂 1 喷 pr.nar tid。
- NS 100mL+ 甲强龙 40mg ivgtt qd。
- NS 100mL+ 泮托拉唑注射液 40mg ivgtt qd。
- 碳酸钙 D_3 片 1 片 po qd。
- 免疫球蛋白针 20g ivgtt qd。
- NS 100mL + 氨溴索 30mg ivgtt bid。

（四）COVID-19 危重型患者医嘱范例

▶ 1. 诊疗医嘱

给予空气隔离、血氧饱和度监测、鼻导管吸氧。

▶ 2. 检查医嘱

- 2019 新型冠状病毒 RNA 测定（三位点）（痰）qd。
- 2019 新型冠状病毒 RNA 测定（三位点）（粪便）qd。
- 血常规、ABO+Rh 血型、尿常规、粪便常规 + OB、常规四项、呼吸道病毒、甲状腺功能、常规心电图、血气分析 + 电解质 + 乳酸 + GS、G/GM 试验、血培养 ONCE。
- 血常规、生化、凝血功能 + D- 二聚体、血气分析 + 乳酸、尿钠肽、心肌酶、血清肌钙蛋白定量、免疫球蛋白 + 补体、细胞因子、痰培养、CRP、PCT 测定 qd。
- 葡萄糖测定 q6h。
- 肝胆胰脾超声、心脏超声、胸部床边摄片、肺部 CT。

▶ 3. 药物医嘱

- 阿比多尔片 200mg po tid。
- 洛匹那韦 / 利托那韦片 2 片 po q12h（或达芦那韦 1 片 po qd）。
- NS 10mL + 甲强龙 40mg iv q12h。

- NS 100mL ＋泮托拉注射液 40mg ivgtt qd。
- 免疫球蛋白针 20g ivgtt qd。
- 胸腺肽针 1.6mg ih biw。
- NS 10mL ＋氨溴索 30mg iv bid。
- NS 50mL ＋异丙肾上腺素 2mg iv-vp ONCE。
- 人血白蛋白 10g ivgtt qd。
- NS 100mL ＋哌拉西林 / 他唑巴坦 4.5g ivgtt q8h。
- 肠内营养混悬液 500mL 鼻饲法 bid。

二、线上咨询诊疗服务流程

（一）线上患者咨询诊疗

浙大一院互联网医院就诊流程

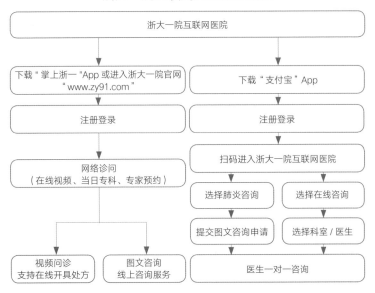

下载"掌上浙一"App 或
进入浙大一院官网"www.zy91.com"

浙大一院互联网医院
（通过支付宝扫码）

如何联系我们
Email: zdyy6616@126.com / zyinternational@163.com

（二）线上医生交流平台

浙大一院国际医生交流平台使用流程

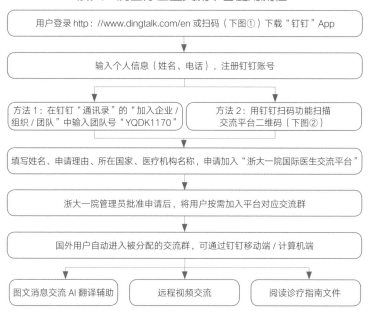

用户登录 http：//www.dingtalk.com/en 或扫码（下图①）下载"钉钉"App

↓

输入个人信息（姓名、电话），注册钉钉账号

↓

方法1：在钉钉"通讯录"的"加入企业/组织/团队"中输入团队号"YQDK1170" ｜ 方法2：用钉钉扫码功能扫描交流平台二维码（下图②）

↓

填写姓名、申请理由、所在国家、医疗机构名称，申请加入"浙大一院国际医生交流平台"

↓

浙大一院管理员批准申请后，将用户按需加入平台对应交流群

↓

国外用户自动进入被分配的交流群，可通过钉钉移动端/计算机端

↓

图文消息交流 AI 翻译辅助 ｜ 远程视频交流 ｜ 阅读诊疗指南文件

备注：具体操作流程可扫码下图③获取。

①扫码下载"钉钉"App ｜ ②交流平台二维码（通过"钉钉"App 扫码）｜ ③操作手册（通过"钉钉"App 扫码）

Part One

Prevention and
Control Management

1 Isolation Area Management

1.1 Fever Clinic

1.1.1 Layout

(1) A relatively independent fever clinic shall be set up in healthcare facilities, with a visible sign showing an exclusive one-way passage to the fever clinic at the entrance of the hospital.

(2) The flow of people shall be guided by the principle of "three zones and two passages": a contaminated zone, a potentially contaminated zone and a clean zone provided and clearly demarcated, and two buffer zones between the contaminated zone and the potentially contaminated zone.

(3) An independent passage shall be equipped for contaminated items; a visual room for one-way delivery of items shall be set up from an office area (potentially contaminated zone) to an isolation ward (contaminated zone).

(4) Appropriate procedures shall be standardized for medical staff to put on and remove their protective equipment, while flowcharts of different zones should be made, full-length mirrors should be provided, and the walking routes must be strictly observed.

(5) Infection prevention and control technicians shall be assigned to supervise the medical staff putting and removing protective equipment so as to prevent contamination.

(6) All items in the contaminated zone that have not been disinfected shall not be removed.

1.1.2 Zone Arrangement

(1) Set up isolated rooms, such as an examination room, a laboratory,

an observation room, a resuscitation room, a hospital pharmacy and a cashier desk.

(2) Set up a pre-examination and triage room for preliminary screening of patients.

(3) Separate diagnosis and treatment zones: those with an epidemiological history and fever and/or respiratory symptoms shall be guided into a zone for suspected patients with COVID-19; those with regular fever but no clear epidemiological history shall be guided into a zone for regular fever patients.

1.1.3 Patient Management

(1) Patients with a fever must wear a surgical mask.

(2) Only patients are allowed to enter the waiting area in order to avoid overcrowding.

(3) The duration of the patients' visit shall be shortened so as to avoid cross infection.

(4) Educate patients and their families about early identification of symptoms and essential prevention measures.

1.1.4 Screening, Admission and Exclusion

(1) All medical workers shall fully understand the epidemiological and clinical features of COVID-19 and screen patients in accordance with the screening criteria (Table 1.1).

(2) Nucleic acid testing (NAT) shall be conducted on those patients who meet the screening criteria for suspected patients.

(3) Patients who do not meet the screening criteria above, are recommended for further evaluation as well as a comprehensive diagnosis, if they do not have a confirmed epidemiological history, but cannot be ruled out from having COVID-19 based on their symptoms, especially through imaging.

(4) Any patient who tests negative shall be re-tested 24 hours later. If a patient has two negative NAT results and negative clinical manifestations, he or she can be ruled out from having COVID-19 and discharged from the hospital. If patients cannot be ruled out from

having COVID-19 infection based on their clinical manifestations, they shall be subjected to additional NAT tests every 24 hours until they are excluded or confirmed.

(5) Those confirmed cases with a positive NAT result shall be admitted and treated collectively based on the severity of their conditions (to the general isolation ward or isolated ICU).

Table 1.1 Screening Criteria for Suspected Cases with COVID-19

Epidemiological history	1. Within 14 days before the onset of COVID-19, the patient has a travel or residence history in high-risk regions or countries. 2. Within 14 days before the onset of COVID-19, the patient has a history of contact with those infected with SARS-CoV-2 (those with a positive NAT result). 3.Within 14 days before the onset of COVID-19, the patient had direct contact with patients with fever or respiratory symptoms in high-risk regions or countries. 4.Disease clustering (2 or more cases with fever and/or respiratory symptoms occur in such places as homes, offices, school classrooms, etc. within 2 weeks)	The patient meets 1 epidemiological history and 2 clinical manifestations	The patient has no epidemiological history and meets 3 clinical manifestations	The patient has no epidemiological history, meets 1-2 clinical manifestations, but cannot be excluded from COVID-19 through imaging
Clinical manifestations	1.The patient has fever and/or respiratory symptoms. 2.The patient has the following CT imaging features of COVID-19: Multiple patchy shadows and interstitial changes occur early, particularly at the lung periphery; the conditions further develop into multiple ground-glass opacities and infiltrates in both lungs. In severe cases, the patient may have lung consolidation and rare pleural effusion. 3.The white blood cell count in the early stage of COVID-19 is normal or decreased, and the lymphocyte count is normal or decreased			
Suspected case diagnosis		Yes	Yes	Expert consultation

1.2 Isolation Ward Area

1.2.1 Scope of Application

The isolation ward area includes an observation ward area, isolation wards, and an isolation ICU area. The building layout and workflow shall meet the relevant requirements of Technique Standard for Isolation in Hospital. Medical providers with negative pressure rooms shall implement standardized management in accordance with relevant requirements. Strictly limit access to isolation wards.

1.2.2 Layout

Please refer to fever clinic.

1.2.3 Ward Requirements

(1) Suspected and confirmed patients shall be separated in different ward areas.

(2) Suspected patients shall be isolated in separated single rooms. Each room shall be equipped with facilities such as a private bathroom and the patient's activity should be confined to the isolation ward.

(3) Confirmed patients can be arranged in the same room with bed spacing no less than 1.2 meters (appx 4 feet). The room shall be equipped with facilities such as a bathroom and the patient's activity must be confined to the isolation ward.

1.2.4 Patient Management

(1) Family visits and nursing shall be declined. Patients should be allowed to have their electronic communication devices to facilitate interactions with loved ones.

(2) Educate patients to help them prevent further spread of COVID-19, and provide instructions on how to wear surgical masks, proper hand washing, cough etiquette, medical observation and home quarantine.

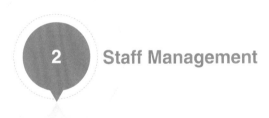

2 Staff Management

2.1 Workflow Management

(1) Before working in a fever clinic and isolation ward, the staff must undergo strict training and examinations to ensure that they know how to put on and remove personal protective equipment. They must pass such examinations before being allowed to work in these wards.

(2) The staff should be divided into different teams. Each team should be limited to a maximum of 4 hours of working in an isolation ward. The teams shall work in the isolation wards (contaminated zones) in different periods.

(3) Arrange treatment, examination and disinfection for each team as a group to reduce the frequency of staff moving in and out of the isolation wards.

(4) Before going off duty, staff must wash themselves and conduct necessary personal hygiene regimens to prevent possible infection of their respiratory tracts and mucosa.

2.2 Health Management

(1) The frontline staff in the isolation areas—including healthcare personnel, medical technicians and property & logistics personnel—shall live in an isolation accommodation and shall not go out without permission.

(2) A nutritious diet shall be provided to improve the immunity of medical staff.

(3) Monitor and record the health status of all staff on the job, conduct health monitoring for frontline staff, including monitoring

body temperature and respiratory symptoms, and help address any psychological and physiological problem that arises with relevant experts.

(4) If the staff have any relevant symptoms such as fever, they shall be isolated immediately and screened with an NAT.

(5) When the frontline staff finish their work in the isolation area and are returning to normal life, they shall first be NAT tested for SARS-CoV-2. If negative, they shall be isolated collectively at a specified area for 14 days before being discharged from medical observation.

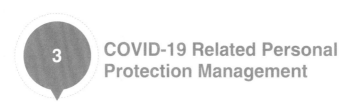

3 COVID-19 Related Personal Protection Management

COVID-19 related personal protection management is shown in Table 1.2.

Table 1.2 COVID-19 Related Personal Protection Management

Protection Level	Protective Equipment	Scope of Application
Level I protection	· Disposable surgical cap · Disposable surgical mask · Work uniform · Disposable latex gloves and/or disposable isolation clothing if necessary	· Pre-examination triage, general outpatient department
Level II protection	· Disposable surgical cap · Medical protective mask (N95) · Work uniform · Disposable medical protective uniform · Disposable latex gloves · Goggles	· Fever outpatient department · Isolation ward area (including isolated ICU) · Non-respiratory specimen examination of suspected/confirmed patients · Imaging examination of suspected/confirmed patients · Cleaning of surgical instruments used with suspected/confirmed patients
Level III protection	· Disposable surgical cap · Medical protective mask (N95) · Work uniform · Disposable medical protective uniform · Disposable latex gloves · Full-face respiratory protective devices or powered air-purifying respirator	· When the staff performs operations such as tracheal intubation, tracheotomy, bronchofibroscope, gastroenterological endoscope, etc., during which, the suspected/confirmed patients may spray or splash respiratory secretions or body fluids/blood · When the staff performs surgery and autopsy for confirmed/suspected patients · When the staff carries out NAT for COVID-19

Notes:
1. All staff at the healthcare facilities must wear surgical masks.
2. All staff working in the emergency department, outpatient department of infectious diseases, outpatient department of respiratory care, department of stomatology, endoscopic examination room (such as gastrointestinal endoscopy, bronchofibroscopy, laryngoscopy, etc.) must upgrade their surgical masks to medical protective masks (N95) based on Level I protection.
3. Staff must wear a protective face screen based on Level II protection while collecting respiratory specimens from suspected/confirmed patients.

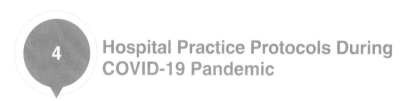

Hospital Practice Protocols During COVID-19 Pandemic

4.1 Guidance on Donning and Doffing Personal Protective Equipment (PPE) to Manage Patients with COVID-19

Protocol for donning PPE (Figure 1-1):

Put on special work clothes and work shoes → Wash hands → Put on a disposable surgical cap → Put on a medical protective mask (N95) → Put on inner disposable nitrile/latex gloves → Put on goggles and protective clothing (note: if wearing protective clothing without foot covers, please also put on separate waterproof boot covers), put on a disposable isolation gown (if required in the specific work zone) and face shield/powered air-purifying respirator (if required in the specific work zone) → Put on outer disposable latex gloves.

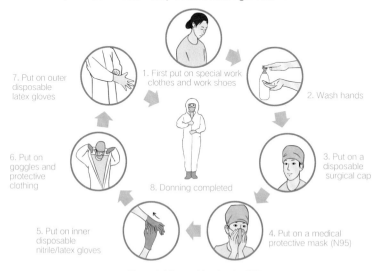

7. Put on outer disposable latex gloves

1. First put on special work clothes and work shoes

2. Wash hands

6. Put on goggles and protective clothing

8. Donning completed

3. Put on a disposable surgical cap

5. Put on inner disposable nitrile/latex gloves

4. Put on a medical protective mask (N95)

Figure 1-1 Protocol for donning PPE

Protocol for doffing PPE (Figure 1-2):

Wash hands and remove visible bodily fluids/blood contaminants on the outer surfaces of both hands → Wash hands and replace outer gloves with new gloves → Remove powered air-purifying respirator or self-priming filter-type full-face mask/mask (if used) → Wash hands → Remove disposable gowns along with outer gloves (if used) → Wash hands and put on outer gloves → Enter Removal Area No.1 → Wash hands and remove protective clothing along with outer gloves (for gloves and protective clothing, turn inside out, while rolling them down) (note: if used, remove the waterproof boot covers with clothing) → Wash hands → Enter Removal Area No.2 → Wash hands and remove goggles → Wash hands and remove the mask → Wash hands and remove the cap → Wash hands and remove inner disposable latex gloves → Wash hands and leave Removal Area No.3 → Wash hands, take a shower, put on clean clothes and enter the clean area.

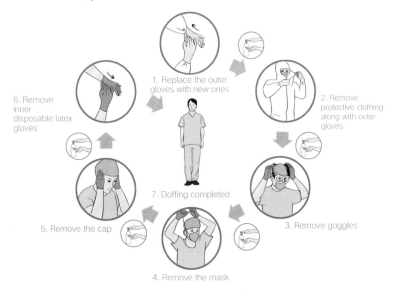

6. Remove inner disposable latex gloves

1. Replace the outer gloves with new ones

2. Remove protective clothing along with outer gloves

7. Doffing completed

5. Remove the cap

3. Remove goggles

4. Remove the mask

Figure 1-2 Protocol for doffing PPE

4.2 Disinfection Procedures for COVID-19 Isolation Ward Area

4.2.1 Disinfection for Floor and Walls

(1) Visible pollutants shall be completely removed before disinfection and handled in accordance with disposal procedures of blood and bodily fluid spills.

(2) Disinfect the floor and walls with 1000 mg/L chlorine-containing disinfectant through floor mopping, spraying or wiping.

(3) Make sure that disinfection is conducted for at least 30 minutes.

(4) Carry out disinfection 3 times a day and repeat the procedure at any time when there is contamination.

4.2.2 Disinfection of Object Surfaces

(1) Visible pollutants should be completely removed before disinfection and handled in accordance with disposal procedures of blood and bodily fluid spills.

(2) Wipe the surfaces of objects with 1000 mg/L chlorine-containing disinfectant or wipes with chlorine; wait for 30 minutes and then rinse with clean water. Perform disinfection procedure 3 times a day. Rrepeat at any time when contamination is suspected.

(3) Wipe cleaner regions first, and then more contaminated regions: First wipe the object surfaces that are not frequently touched, and then the object surfaces that are frequently touched (once the surface of an object is wiped clean, replace the used wipe with a new one).

4.2.3 Air Disinfection

(1) Plasma air sterilizers can be used and continuously run for air disinfection in an environment with human activity.

(2) If there are no plasma air sterilizers, use ultraviolet lamps for 1 hour each time and 3 times a day.

4.2.4 Disposal of Fecal Matter and Sewage

(1) Before being discharged into the municipal drainage system, fecal

matter and sewage must be disinfected by treating with chlorine-containing disinfectant (for the initial treatment, the active chlorine must be more than 40 mg/L). Make sure the disinfection time is at least 1.5 hours.

(2) The concentration of total residual chlorine in the disinfected sewage should reach 10 mg/L.

4.3 Disposal Procedures for Blood/Bodily Fluids/ Vomit etc. of Patients with COVID-19

4.3.1 For Spills of a Small Volume ($<$ 10 mL) of Blood/Bodily Fluids

(1) Option 1: The spills should be covered with chlorine-containing disinfecting wipes (containing 5000 mg/L active chlorine) and carefully removed, and then the surfaces of the object should be wiped twice with chlorine-containing disinfecting wipes (containing 5000 mg/L active chlorine).

(2) Option 2: Carefully remove the spills with disposable absorbent materials such as gauze, wipes, etc., which have been soaked in 5000 mg/ L chlorine-containing disinfecting solution.

4.3.2 For Spills of a Large Volume ($>$ 10 mL) of Blood/Bodily Fluids

(1) First, place signs to indicate the presence of a spill.

(2) Perform disposal procedures according to option 1 or 2 described below.

① Option 1: Absorb the spilled fluids for 30 minutes with a clean absorbent towel (containing peroxyacetic acid that can absorb up to 1 L of liquid per towel), and then clean the contaminated area after removing the pollutants.

① Option 2: Completely cover the spill with disinfectant powder or bleach powder containing water-absorbing ingredients or completely cover it with disposable water-absorbing materials, and then pour a sufficient amount of 10,000 mg/L chlorine-containing disinfectant onto the water-absorbing material (or cover with a dry towel which will be subjected to high-level disinfection). Leave for at least 30 minutes before carefully removing the spills.

(3) Fecal matter, secretions, vomit, etc. from patients shall be collected into special containers and disinfected for 2 hours by a 20,000 mg/L chlorine-containing disinfectant at a spill-to-disinfectant ratio of 1 : 2.

(4) After removing the spills, disinfect the surfaces of the polluted environment or objects.

(5) The containers that hold the contaminants can be soaked and disinfected with 5000 mg/L chlorine-containing disinfectant for 30 minutes and then cleaned.

(6) The collected pollutants should be disposed of as medical waste.

(7) The used items should be put into double-layer medical waste bags and disposed of as medical waste.

4.4 Disinfection of COVID-19 Related Reusable Medical Devices

4.4.1 Disinfection of Powered Air-Purifying Respirator

The procedures for disinfection of powered air-purifying respirator are shown in Figure 1-3.

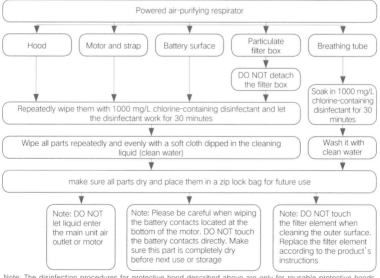

Note: The disinfection procedures for protective hood described above are only for reusable protective hoods (excluding disposable protective hoods).

Figure 1-3 Disinfection of powered air-purifying respirator

4.4.2 Cleaning and Disinfection Procedures for Digestive Endoscopy and Bronchofibroscopy

(1) Soak the endoscope and reusable valves in 0.23% peroxyacetic acid (confirm the concentration of the disinfectant before use to make sure it will be effective).

(2) Connect the perfusion line of each channel of the endoscope, inject 0.23% peroxyacetic acid liquid into the line with a 50 mL syringe until fully filled, and wait for 5 minutes.

(3) Detach the perfusion line and wash each cavity and valve of the endoscope with a disposable special cleaning brush.

(4) Put the valves into an ultrasonic oscillator containing enzyme to oscillate it. Connect the perfusion line of each channel with the endoscope. Inject 0.23% peroxyacetic acid into the line with a 50 mL syringe and flush the line continuously for 5 minutes. Inject air to dry it for 1 minute.

(5) Inject clean water into the line with a 50 mL syringe and flush the line continuously for 3 minutes. Inject air to dry it for 1 minute.

(6) Perform a leakage test on the endoscope.

(7) Put in an automatic endoscopic washing and disinfection machine. Set a high level of disinfection for treatment.

(8) Send the devices to the disinfection supply center to undergo sterilization with ethylene oxide.

4.4.3 Pre-treatment of Other Reusable Medical Devices

(1) If there are no visible pollutants, soak the device in 1000 mg/L chlorine-containing disinfectant for at least 30 minutes.

(2) If there are any visible pollutants, soak the device in 5000 mg/L chlorine-containing disinfectant for at least 30 minutes.

(3) After drying, pack and fully enclose the devices and send them to the disinfection supply center.

4.5 Disinfection Procedures for Infectious Fabrics of Suspected or Confirmed Patients

4.5.1 Infectious Fabrics

(1) Clothes, bed sheets, bed covers and pillowcases used by patients.

(2) Bed curtains in ward area.

(3) Floor towels used for environmental cleaning.

4.5.2 Collection Methods

(1) Pack the fabrics into a disposable water-soluble plastic bag and seal the bag with matching cable ties.

(2) Pack this bag into another plastic bag, seal the bag with cable ties in a gooseneck fashion.

(3) Pack the plastic bag into a yellow fabric bag and seal the bag with cable ties.

(4) Attach a special infection label and the department name. Send the bag to the laundry room.

4.5.3 Storage and Washing

(1) Infectious fabrics should be separated from other infectious fabrics (non-COVID-19) and washed in a dedicated washing machine.

(2) Wash and disinfect these fabrics with chlorine-containing disinfectant at 90°C for at least 30 minutes.

4.5.4 Disinfection of Transport Tools

(1) Special transport tools should be used specifically for transporting infectious fabrics.

(2) The tools shall be disinfected immediately after being used for transporting infectious fabrics.

(3) The transport tools should be wiped with chlorine-containing disinfectant (with 1000 mg/L chlorine). Leave disinfectant for 30 minutes before wiping the tools clean with clean water.

4.6 Disposal Procedures for COVID-19 Related Medical Waste

(1) All waste generated from suspected or confirmed patients shall be disposed of as medical waste.

(2) Put the medical waste into a double-layer medical waste bag, seal the bag with cable ties in a gooseneck fashion and spray the bag with

1000 mg/L chlorine-containing disinfectant.

(3) Put sharp objects into a special plastic box, seal the box and spray the box with 1000 mg/L chlorine-containing disinfectant.

(4) Put the bagged waste into a medical waste transfer box, attach a special infection label, fully enclose the box and transfer it.

(5) Transfer the waste to a temporary storage point for medical waste along a specified route at a fixed time point and store the waste separately at a fixed location.

(6) The medical waste shall be collected and disposed of by an approved medical waste disposal provider.

4.7 Procedures for Taking Remedial Actions against Occupational Exposure to COVID-19

Procedures for taking remedial actions against occupational exposure to COVID-19 are shown in Figure 1-4.

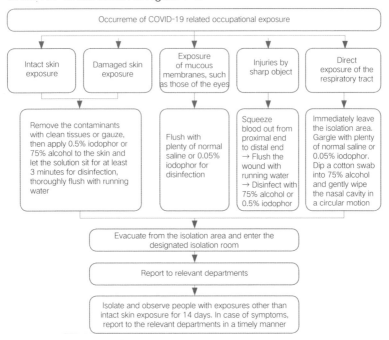

Figure 1-4 Procedures for taking remedial actions against occupational exposure to COVID-19

(1) Skin exposure: The skin is directly contaminated by a large amount of visible bodily fluids, blood, secretions or fecal matter from the patient.

(2) Mucous membrane exposure: Mucous membranes, such as those of the eyes, and the respiratory tract, are directly contaminated by visible bodily fluids, blood, secretions or fecal matter from the patient.

(3) Sharp object injury: piercing of the body by sharp objects that are directly exposed to the patient's bodily fluids, blood, secretions or fecal matter.

(4) Direct exposure of the respiratory tract: falling off of a mask, exposing the mouth or the nose to a confirmed patient (less than 1 meter) who is not wearing a mask.

4.8 Surgical Operations for Suspected or Confirmed Patients

4.8.1 Requirements for Operation Rooms and Staff PPE

(1) Arrange the patients in a negative pressure operating room. Verify the temperature, humidity and air pressure in the operation room.

(2) Prepare all required items for the operation and use disposable surgical items if possible.

(3) All surgical personnel (including surgeons, anesthesiologists, hand-washing nurses, and charge nurses in operating rooms) should put on their PPE in the buffer room before entering the operating room: Put on double caps, medical protective masks (N95), medical goggles (if needed), medical protective clothing, boot covers, latex gloves, and powered air-purifying respirators.

(4) The surgeons and the hand-washing nurses should wear disposable sterile operating clothes and sterile gloves in addition to the PPE as mentioned above.

(5) Patients should wear disposable caps and disposable surgical masks depending on their situation.

(6) The charge nurses in the buffer room are responsible for delivering items from the buffer area to the negative pressure operating room.

(7) During the operation, the buffer room and the operating room shall be tightly closed, and the operation must be carried out only if the

operation room is under negative pressure.

(8) Irrelevant personnel shall be excluded from entering the operating room.

4.8.2 Procedures for Final Disinfection

(1) Medical waste shall be disposed of as COVID-19 related medical waste.

(2) Reusable medical devices shall be disinfected according to the disinfection procedures of COVID-19 related reusable medical devices.

(3) Medical fabrics shall be disinfected and disposed of according to the disinfection procedures for COVID-19 related infectious fabrics.

(4) Surfaces of objects (instruments and devices including device table, operating table, operating bed, etc.).

① Visible blood/bodily fluid pollutants shall be completely removed before disinfection (handled in accordance with disposal procedures of blood and bodily fluid spills).

② All surfaces shall be wiped with a disinfectant containing 1000 mg/L chlorine and allowed to sit for 30 minutes with the disinfectant.

(5) Floor and walls:

① Visible blood/bodily fluid pollutants shall be completely removed before disinfection (handled in accordance with disposal procedures of blood and bodily fluid spills).

② All surfaces shall be wiped with a disinfectant containing 1000 mg/L chlorine and allowed to sit for 30 minutes with the disinfectant.

(6) Indoor air: Turn off the fan filter unit (FFU). Disinfect the air by irradiation with ultraviolet lamp for at least 1 hour. Turn on the FFU to purify the air automatically for at least 2 hours.

4.9 Procedures for Handling Bodies of Deceased Suspected or Confirmed Patients

(1) Staff PPE: The staff must make sure they are fully protected by wearing work clothes, disposable surgical caps, disposable gloves and thick rubber gloves with long sleeves, medical disposable protective clothing, medical protective masks (N95) or powered air purifying

respirators (PAPRs), protective face shields, work shoes or rubber boots, waterproof boot covers, waterproof aprons or waterproof isolation gowns, etc.

(2) Corpse care: Fill all openings or wounds the patient may have, such as mouth, nose, ears, anus and tracheotomy openings, by using cotton balls or gauze dipped in 3000-5000 mg/L chlorine-containing disinfectant or 0.5% peroxyacetic acid.

(3) Wrapping: Wrap the corpse with a double-layer cloth sheet soaked with disinfectant, and pack it into a double-layer, sealed, leak-proof corpse wrapping sheet soaked with chlorine containing disinfectant.

(4) The corpse shall be transferred by the staff in the isolation ward of the hospital via the contaminated area to the special elevator, out of the ward, and then directly transported to a specified location for cremation by a special vehicle as soon as possible.

(5) Final disinfection: Disinfect the wards and the special elevators.

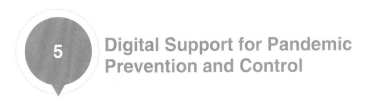

5 Digital Support for Pandemic Prevention and Control

5.1 Lower the Risk of Cross Infection by Patients Receiving Medical Care

(1) Guide the public to get access to non-emergency services such as chronic diseases treatment online so as to decrease the number of visitors in healthcare facilities, and to minimize the risk of cross infection.

(2) Patients who must visit healthcare facilities should make an appointment through Internet portals, which provide necessary guidance on transportation, parking, arrival time, protective measures, triage information, indoor navigation, etc. Comprehensive information of patients are supposed to be collected online in advance to improve the efficiency of diagnoses and treatments, therefore the duration of the patient's visit in the hospital can be shortened.

(3) Encourage patients to take full advantage of digital self-service devices to avoid contact with others so as to lower the risk of cross infection.

5.2 Lower Work Intensity and Infection Risk of Medical Staff

(1) Collect shared knowledge and experience of experts through remote consultation and multidisciplinary team (MDT) to offer the optimum therapeutics for difficult and complicated cases.

(2) Take mobile and remote rounds to lower unnecessary exposure risk and work intensity of medical staff while saving protective supplies.

(3) Access the patients' latest health conditions electronically through

health QR codes (note: Everyone is required to obtain a GREEN code (healthy code) through the health QR system to travel around the city) and online epidemiological questionnaires in advance to provide triage guidance to the patients, especially those with fever or suspected cases, while effectively preventing the risk of infection.

(4) Electronic health records of patients in fever clinics and the CT imaging artificial intelligence (AI) system for COVID-19 can help reduce work intensity, quickly identify highly-suspected cases and avoid missed diagnoses.

5.3 Rapid Responses to Emergency Needs of COVID-19 Containment

(1) Basic digital resources required by a cloud-based hospital system allow for immediate usage of the information systems needed for emergency responses to the epidemic, such as the digital systems equipped for newly established fever clinics, fever observation rooms and isolation wards.

(2) Utilize the hospital information system based on the Internet infrastructure frame to conduct online training for healthcare workers and one-click deployment system, and to facilitate the operation and support engineers to perform remote maintenance and new functions update for healthcare.

【FAHZU Internet + Hospital: A Model for Online Healthcare】
Since the outbreak of COVID-19, FAHZU Internet + Hospital has been quickly shifted to offer online healthcare through Zhejiang's Online Medical Platform with 24-hour free online consultation, providing telemedicine service to patients in China and even around the world. Patients are provided an access to the first-rate medical services of FAHZU at home, which lowers the risk of transmission and cross infection resulting from their visits to the hospital. As of March 14, 2020, over 10,000 people have used the FAHZU Internet+ Hospital online service.

· **Instructions for Zhejiang Online Medical Platform**
① Download Alipay App.
② Open Alipay (Mainland Version) and find "Zhejiang Provincial Online Medical Platform".
③ Choose a hospital (The First Affiliated Hospital, Zhejiang University School of Medicine).
④ Post your question and wait for a doctor to respond.
⑤ A notification will pop up when a doctor replies. Then open Alipay and click [Friends]-[Lifestyle].
⑥ Click [Zhejiang Online Medical Platform] to see more details and start your consultation.

【Establishing the International Medical Expert Communication Platform of the First Affiliated Hospital, Zhejiang University School of Medicine】

Due to the spread of the COVID-19 pandemic, The First Affiliated Hospital, Zhejiang University School of Medicine (FAHZU) and Alibaba jointly established the International Medical Expert Communication Platform of FAHZU with an aim to improve the quality of medical care and treatment and to promote sharing of global information resource. The platform allows medical experts all over the world to connect and share their invaluable experience in the fight against such an pandemic through instant messaging with real-time translation, remote video conferencing, etc.

· **Instructions on the International Medical Expert Communication Platform of The First Affiliated Hospital, Zhejiang University School of Medicine**
① Visit www.dingtalk.com/en to download DingTalk App.
② Sign up with your personal information (name and phone number) and log in.
③ Apply to join the International Medical Expert Communication Platform of FAHZU.
Method 1: Join by team code. Select "Contacts"-"Join Team"-"Join by Team Code", and then enter the Input ID, "YQDK1170".

Method 2: Join by scanning the QR code of the International Medical Expert Communication Platform of FAHZU.

④ Fill out your information to join. Enter your name, country and medical institution.

⑤ Join the FAHZU group chat after the administrator approves.

⑥ After joining the group chat, medical staff can send instant messages assisted by AI translation, receive remote video guidance, and have an access to medical treatment guidelines.

Part Two

Diagnosis and Treatment

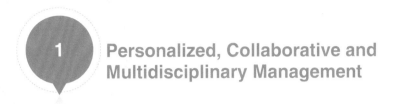

Personalized, Collaborative and Multidisciplinary Management

FAHZU is a designated hospital for patients with COVID-19, especially severe and critically ill ones, whose condition changes rapidly, often with multiple organs infected, requiring support from the multidisciplinary team (MDT). Since the outbreak of COVID-19, FAHZU has established an expert team composed of doctors from the Departments of Infectious Diseases, Respiratory Medicine, ICU, Laboratory Medicine, Radiology, Ultrasound, Pharmacy, Traditional Chinese Medicine, Psychology, Respiratory Therapy, Rehabilitation, Nutrition, Nursing, etc. A comprehensive multidisciplinary diagnosis and treatment mechanism has been established in which doctors both inside and outside isolation wards can discuss about patients' conditions every day via video conference. This allows for them to determine scientific, integrated and customized treatment strategies for every severe and critically ill patient.

Sound decision-making is the key to MDT discussion. During the discussion, experts from different departments focus on issues from their specialized fields as well as critical issues to diagnoses and treatment. The final treatment solution would be determined by experienced experts through various discussions with different opinions and advice.

Systematic analysis is at the core of MDT discussion. Elderly patients with underlying health conditions are prone to becoming critically ill. While closely monitoring the progression of COVID-19, the patients' basic status, complications and daily examination results should be analyzed comprehensively to see how the disease will progress. It is necessary to intervene in advance to stop the disease from deteriorating and to take proactive measures such as antivirals, oxygen therapy, and nutritional support.

The goal of MDT discussion is to achieve personalized treatment. The treatment plan should be adjusted to each person when considering the differences among individuals, courses of disease, and patient types.

Our experience is that MDT collaboration can greatly improve the effectiveness of the diagnosis and treatment of COVID-19.

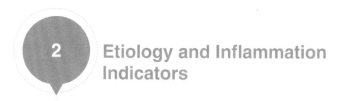

2 Etiology and Inflammation Indicators

2.1 Detection of SARS-CoV-2 Nucleic Acid

2.1.1 Specimen Collection

Appropriate specimens, collection methods and collection timing are all important to improve detection sensitivity. Specimen types include: upper airway specimens (pharyngeal swabs, nasal swabs, and nasopharyngeal secretions), lower airway specimens (sputum, airway secretions, bronchoalveolar lavage fluid), blood, feces, urine and conjunctival secretions. Sputum and other lower respiratory tract specimens have a high positive rate of nucleic acids and should be collected preferentially. SARS-CoV-2 preferentially proliferates in type II alveolar cells (AT2) and peak of viral shedding appears 3 to 5 days after the onset of COVID-19. Therefore, if the nucleic acid test is negative at the beginning, samples should continue to be collected and tested on subsequent days and more patients would be tested positive.

2.1.2 Nucleic Acid Detection

Nucleic acid testing is the first-choice method for diagnosing SARS-CoV-2 infection. According to the kit instructions, the testing procedure is as follows: Specimens are pre-processed, and the virus is lysed to extract nucleic acids. The three specific genes of SARS-CoV-2, namely the open reading frame 1a/b (ORF1a/b), nucleocapsid protein (N), and envelope protein (E) genes, are then amplified by real-time quantitative PCR technology. The amplified genes are detected by fluorescence intensity. Criteria of positive nucleic acid results are: ORF1a/b gene is positive, and/or N gene/E gene is positive.

The combined detection of nucleic acids from multiple types of specimens can improve the diagnostic accuracy. Among patients with confirmed positive nucleic acid in the respiratory tract, about 30%–40% of these patients have detected viral nucleic acid in the blood and about 50%–60% of patients have detected viral nucleic acid in feces. However, the positive rate of nucleic acid testing in urine samples is quite low. Combined testing with specimens from the respiratory tract, feces, blood and other types of specimens is helpful for improving the diagnostic sensitivity of suspected cases, monitoring treatment efficacy and the management of post-discharge isolation measures.

2.2 Virus Isolation and Culture

Virus culture must be performed in a laboratory with qualified biosafety level 3 (BSL-3). The process is briefly described as follows: Fresh samples of the patient's sputum, feces, etc. are obtained and inoculated on Vero-E6 cells for virus culture. The cytopathic effect (CPE) is observed after 96 hours. Detection of viral nucleic acid in the culture medium indicates a successful culture. Virus titer measurement: After diluting the virus stock concentration by a factor of 10 in series, 50% tissue culture intertions dose ($TCID_{50}$) is determined by the micro-cytopathic method. Otherwise, viral viability is determined by plaque forming unit (PFU).

2.3 Detection of Serum Antibody

Specific antibodies are produced after SARS-CoV-2 infection. Serum antibody determination methods include colloidal gold immunochromatography, enzyme-linked immunosorbent assay (ELISA), chemiluminescence immunoassay, etc. Positive serum-specific immunoglobulin M (IgM), or specific IgG antibody titer in the recovery phase no less than 4 times higher than that in the acute phase, can be used as diagnostic criteria for suspected patients with negative nucleic acid detection. During follow-up monitoring, IgM is detectable 10 days after symptom onset and IgG is detectable 12 days after symptom onset. The viral load gradually decreases with an increase of serum antibody level.

2.4 Detecting Indicators of Inflammatory Response

It is recommended to conduct tests of C-reactive protein (CRP), procalcitonin (PCT), ferritin, D-dimer, total and subpopulations of lymphocytes, interleukin-4 (IL-4), IL-6, IL-10, tumor necrosis factor- α (TNF- α), interferon- γ (INF- γ) and other indicators of inflammation and immune status, which can help evaluate clinical progress, alert severe and critical tendencies, and provide a basis for the formulation of treatment strategies.

Most patients with COVID-19 have a normal level of PCT with significantly increased levels of CRP. A rapid and significantly elevated CRP level indicates a possibility of secondary infection. D-dimer levels are significantly elevated in severe cases, which is a potential risk factor for poor prognosis. Patients with a low total number of lymphocytes at the beginning of COVID-19 generally have a poor prognosis. Severe patients have a progressively decreased number of peripheral blood lymphocytes. The expression levels of IL-6 and IL-10 in severe patients are greatly increased. Monitoring the levels of IL-6 and IL-10 is helpful to assess the risk of progression to a severe condition.

2.5 Detection of Secondary Bacterial or Fungal Infections

Severe and critically ill patients are vulnerable to secondary bacterial or fungal infections. Qualified specimens should be collected from the infection site for bacterial or fungal culture. If secondary lung infection is suspected, sputum coughed from deep in the lungs, tracheal aspirates, broncho-alveolar lavage fluid, and brush specimens should be collected for culture. Timely blood culture should be performed in patients with high fever. Blood cultures drawn from peripheral venous or catheters should be performed in patients with suspected sepsis who had an indwelling catheter. It is recommended that they take blood G test and GM test at least twice a week in addition to fungal culture.

2.6 Laboratory Safety

Biosafety protective measures should be determined based on different risk levels of experimental process. Personal protection should be taken in accordance with BSL-3 laboratory protection requirements for specimen collection of the respiratory tract, nucleic acid detection and virus culture operations. Personal protection following BSL-2 laboratory protection requirement should be carried out for biochemical, immunological tests and other routine laboratory tests. Specimens should be transported in special transport tanks and boxes that meet biosafety requirements. All laboratory waste should be strictly autoclaved.

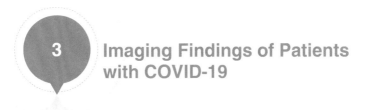

Imaging Findings of Patients with COVID-19

Thoracic imaging is of great value in the diagnosis of COVID-19, monitoring of therapeutic efficacy, and patient discharge assessment. A high-resolution CT is highly preferable. Portable chest X-rays are helpful for critically ill patients who are immobile. CT for baseline evaluation of patients with COVID-19 is usually performed on the day of admission, or if ideal therapeutic efficacy is not reached, it can be re-performed after 2 to 3 days. If symptoms are stable or improved after treatment, the chest CT scan can be reviewed after 5 to 7 days. Daily routine portable chest X-rays are recommended for critically ill patients.

COVID-19 at the early stage often presents with multifocal patchy shadows or ground glass opacities located in the lung periphery, subpleural area, and both lower lobes on chest CT scans. The long axis of the lesion is mostly parallel to the pleura. Interlobular septal thickening and intralobular interstitial thickening, displaying as subpleural reticulation namely a "crazy paving" pattern, is observed in some ground glass opacities. A small number of cases may show solitary, local lesions, or nodular/patchy lesion distributed consistent with bronchus with peripheral ground glass opacities changes. Disease progression mostly occurs in the course of 7 to 10 days, with enlarged and increased density of the lesions compared with previous images, and consolidated lesions with air bronchogram sign. Critically ill cases may show further expanded consolidation, with the whole lung density showing increased opacity, sometimes known as a "white lung". After the condition is relieved, the ground glass opacities can be completely absorbed, and some consolidation lesions will leave fibrotic stripes or subpleural reticulation. Patients with multiple lobular involvement, especially those with expanded lesions should be observed for disease exacerbation. Those with typical CT pulmonary manifestations should be isolated and undergo continuous nucleic acid tests even if the nucleic acid test of SARS-CoV-2 is negative (Figure 2-1).

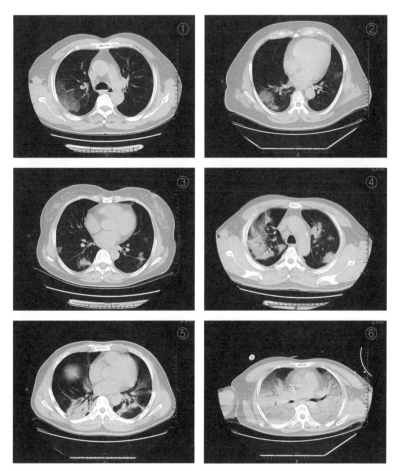

Figure 2-1 Typical CT features of patients with COVID-19. ① & ② patchy ground glass opacities; ③ nodules and patchy exudation; ④ & ⑤ multifocal consolidation lesions; ⑥ diffuse consolidation, "white lung"

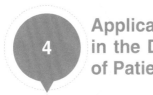

Application of Bronchoscopy in the Diagnosis and Management of Patients with COVID-19

Flexible bronchoscopy is versatile, easy to use, and well tolerated in mechanically ventilated patients with COVID-19. Its applications include the following.

(1) Collection of respiratory specimens from the lower respiratory tract (i.e., sputum, endotracheal aspirate, bronchoalveolar lavage) for SARS-CoV-2 or other pathogens guides the selection of appropriate antimicrobials, which may lead to clinical benefits. Our experience indicates that lower respiratory tract specimens are more likely to be positive for SARS-CoV-2 than upper respiratory tract specimens.

(2) Can be used for localization of the site of bleeding, cessation of hemoptysis, sputum or blood clots removal; if the site of bleeding is identified by bronchoscopy, local injection of cold saline, epinephrine, vasopressin, or fibrin as well as laser treatment can be performed via the bronchoscope.

(3) Assist in the establishment of artificial airways, and guide tracheal intubation or percutaneous tracheotomy.

(4) Drugs such as infusion of IFN-α and N-acetylcysteine can be administered via the bronchoscope.

Bronchoscopic views of extensive bronchial mucosal hyperemia, swelling, mucus-like secretions in the lumen and jelly-like sputum blocking the airway in critically ill patients are shown in Figure 2-2.

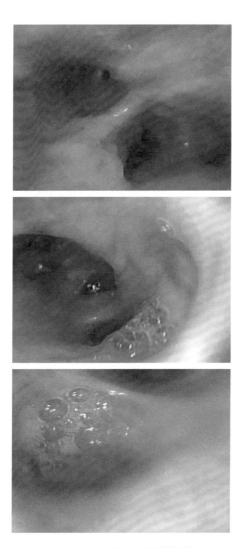

Figure 2-2 Bronchoscopic manifestations of patients with COVID-19: extensive bronchial mucosa swelling and congestion; large amounts of mucus secretions in the lumen

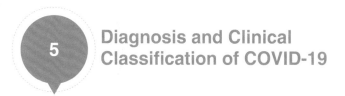

Diagnosis and Clinical Classification of COVID-19

Early diagnosis, treatment and isolation should be carried out whenever possible. Dynamic monitoring of lung imaging, oxygenation index and cytokine levels are helpful for early identification of patients who may develop into severe and critical cases. A positive result of the nucleic acid of SARS-CoV-2 is the gold standard for the diagnosis of COVID-19. However, considering the possibility of false negatives in nucleic acid detection, suspected patients who show typical manifestations in the CT scans can be treated as confirmed cases even if the nucleic acid test is negative. Isolation and continuous tests of multiple specimens should be carried out in such cases.

The diagnostic criteria follow Protocols for the Diagnosis and Treatment of COVID-19. A confirmed case is based on epidemiological history (including cluster transmission), clinical manifestations (fever and respiratory symptoms), lung imaging, and results of SARS-CoV-2 nucleic acid detection and serum-specific antibodies.

Clinical Classifications include the follows.

(1) Mild cases. The clinical symptoms are mild and no pneumonia manifestations can be found in imaging.

(2) Moderate cases. Patients have symptoms such as fever and respiratory tract symptoms, etc., and pneumonia manifestations can be seen in imaging.

(3) Severe cases. Adults who meet any of the following criteria should be treated as severe cases: respiratory rate$\geq$30 breaths/min; oxygen saturation$\leq$93% at a rest state; partial pressure of oxygen in arterial blood (PaO_2)/fraction of inspired oxygen (FiO_2)$\leq$300 mmHg (1 mmHg $\approx$ 0.133 kPa); patients with over 50% lesions progression

within 24 to 48 hours in lung imaging.

(4) Critical cases. Those meeting any of the following criteria should be monitored and receive treatment in the ICU: occurrence of respiratory failure requiring mechanical ventilation; presence of shock; other organ failure.

Critical cases are further divided into early, middle and late stages according to the oxygenation index and compliance of the respiratory system.

● Early stage: 100 mmHg<oxygenation index≤150 mmHg; compliance of respiratory system≥30 mL/cmH$_2$O (1 cmH$_2$O ≈ 0.098 kPa); without organ failure other than the lungs. The patient has a great chance of recovery through active antiviral, anti-cytokine storm, and supportive treatment.

● Middle stage: 60 mmHg<oxygenation index≤100 mmHg; 15 mL/cmH$_2$O≤compliance of respiratory system<30 mL/cmH$_2$O; may be complicated with mild or moderate dysfunction of other organs.

● Late stage: oxygenation index≤60 mmHg; compliance of respiratory system<15 mL/cmH$_2$O; diffuse consolidation of both lungs that requires the use of ECMO; or failure of other vital organs. The mortality risk is significantly increased.

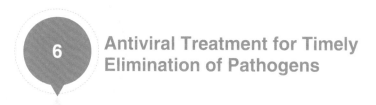

6 Antiviral Treatment for Timely Elimination of Pathogens

An early antiviral treatment can reduce the incidence of severe and critical cases. Although there is no clinical evidence for effective antiviral drugs, currently the antiviral strategies based on the characteristics of SARS-CoV-2 are adopted according to Protocols for Diagnosis and Treatment of COVID-19.

6.1 Antiviral Treatment

At FAHZU, lopinavir/ritonavir (2 capsules, po q12h) combined with Arbidol (200 mg po tid) was applied as the basic regimen. From the treatment experience of 49 patients in our hospital, the average time to achieve negative viral nucleic acid test for the first time was 12 days (95% CI: 8–15 days). The duration of negative nucleic acid test result (negative for more than 2 times consecutively with an interval longer than or equal to 24 hours) was 13.5 days (95% CI: 9.5–17.5 days).

If the basic regimen is not effective, chloroquine phosphate can be used on adults between 18 and 65 years old (weight≥50 kg: 500 mg bid; weight<50 kg: 500 mg bid for the first 2 days, 500 mg qd for the following 5 days).

Interferon nebulization is recommended in Protocols for Diagnosis and Treatment of COVID-19. We recommend that it should be performed in negative-pressure wards rather than general wards due to the possibility of aerosol transmission.

Darunavir/cobicistat has some degree of antiviral activity in viral suppression test *in vitro*, based on the treatment experience of AIDS patients, and the adverse events are relatively mild. For patients who are intolerant to lopinavir/ritonavir, darunavir/cobicistat (1 tablet qd) or favipiravir (starting dose of 1600 mg followed by 600 mg tid) is an alternative option after the ethical review. Simultaneous use of 3 or more antiviral drugs is not recommended.

6.2 Course of Treatment

The treatment course of chloroquine phosphate should be no more than 7 days. The treatment course of other regimens has not been determined and is usually around 2 weeks. Antiviral drugs should be stopped if nucleic acid test results from sputum specimens remain negative for more than 3 times.

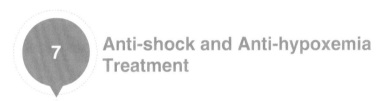

Anti-shock and Anti-hypoxemia Treatment

During the progression from the severe stage to critically ill stage, patients may develop severe hypoxemia, cytokine storm and secondary infections that might develop into shock, tissue perfusion disorders, and even multiple organ failure. Treatment is aimed at incentive removal and fluid resuscitation. The artificial liver support system (ALSS) and blood purification can effectively diminish inflammatory mediators and cytokine storm and prevent the incidence of shock, hypoxemia and acute respiratory distress syndrome.

7.1 Usage of Glucocorticoids When Necessary

Appropriate and short-term use of corticosteroids to inhibit cytokine storm and to prevent disease progression should be considered for patients with severe COVID-19 as early as possible. However, a high dose of glucocorticoids should be avoided due to adverse events and complications.

7.1.1 Indications for Corticosteroids

(1) For those in severe and critically ill stages.

(2) For those with persistent high fever (temperature above 39℃).

(3) For those whose computerized tomography (CT) scans demonstrate patchy ground-glass attenuation or more than 30% area of the lungs are involved.

(4) For those whose CT scans demonstrate rapid progression (more than 50% area involved in pulmonary CT images within 48 hours).

(5) For those whose IL-6 is more than or equal to 5 ULN.

7.1.2 Application of Corticosteroids

Initial routine methylprednisolone at a dose of 0.75 to 1.5 mg/kg intravenously once or twice a day is recommended. However, methylprednisolone at a dose of 40 mg q12h can be considered for patients with falling body temperature or for patients with significantly increased cytokines under routine doses of steroid. Even methylprednisolone at a dose of 40 to 80 mg q12h can be considered for critical cases. Closely monitor body temperature, oxygen saturation, blood routine, C-reactive protein, cytokines, biochemical profile, blood sugar levels and lung CT every 2 to 3 days during the treatment as necessary. The dosage of methylprednisolone should be halved every 3 to 5 days if medical conditions of patients are improved, the body temperature normalizes, or involved lesions on CT are significantly absorbed. Oral methylprednisolone (Medrol) once a day is recommended when the intravenous dose is reduced to 20 mg per day. The course of corticosteroids is not defined; some experts have suggested ceasing corticosteroids treatment when patients are nearly recovered.

7.1.3 Special Considerations during Treatment

(1) Screening of TB by T-SPOT assay, HBV and HCV by antibody assay should be performed before corticosteroid therapy.

(2) Proton pump inhibitors could be considered to prevent complications.

(3) Blood glucose should be monitored. High blood glucose should be treated with insulin when necessary.

(4) Low serum potassium should be corrected.

(5) Liver function should be closely monitored.

(6) Traditional Chinese medicine may be considered for patients who are sweating.

(7) Sedative-hypnotics can be administered temporarily for patients with sleep disorder.

7.2 Artificial Liver Treatment for Suppression of Cytokine Storm

The artificial liver support system (ALSS) can conduct plasma exchange, adsorption, perfusion, and filtration of inflammatory mediators such as endotoxins and harmful metabolic substances of small or medium molecular weight. It cannot only provide serum albumin, coagulation factors, balance fluid volume water, electrolytes and acid-base ratio, and manifest anti-cytokine storm, shock, lung inflammation, etc., but also help to improve multiple organ functions including the liver and the kidney. Thus, it can improve the success rate of treatment and reduce the mortality of severe patients.

7.2.1 Indications for ALSS

Patients who meet (1) + (2) , or patients who meet (3) need ALSS.

(1) Serum inflammatory indicator (such as IL-6) level rises to 5 ULN or over 5 ULN, or the rising rate is no less than 1 time per day.

(2) Involved area of pulmonary CT or X-ray images is no less than 10% progression per day.

(3) ALSS is required for the treatment of underlying diseases.

7.2.2 Contraindications

There is no absolute contraindication in the treatment of critically ill patients. However, ALSS should be avoided in the following situations.

(1) Severe active bleeding disease or disseminated intravascular coagulation.

(2) Highly allergic to blood components or drugs used in the treatment process such as plasma, heparin and protamine.

(3) Acute cerebrovascular diseases or severe head injury.

(4) Chronic cardiac failure, cardiac functional classification are no less than grade III .

(5) Uncontrolled hypotension and shock.

(6) Severe arrhythmia.

Plasma exchange combined with plasma adsorption or dual plasma molecular adsorption, perfusion, and filtration is recommended if the patients follow the indications. Over 2000 mL of plasma should be exchanged when ALSS is performed. With plasma resources being limited, hemoperfusion and hemofiltration can be adopted. Detailed operating procedures can be found in the Expert Consensus on the Application of Artificial Liver Blood Purification System in the Treatment of Severe and Critical III COVID-19 Patients.

ALSS significantly shortens the period that critically ill patients stay in ICU. Typically, the levels of serum cytokines such as IL-2/IL-4/IL-6/TNF-α are remarkably decreased, while oxygen saturation is significantly improved after ALSS.

7.3 Oxygen Therapy for Hypoxemia

Hypoxemia can be presented due to impaired respiratory functions by COVID-19. Oxygen supplementation treatment can correct hypoxemia, and relieve secondary organ damage caused by respiratory distress and hypoxemia.

7.3.1 Oxygen Therapy

(1) Continual monitoring of oxygen saturation during oxygen therapy.

Some patients do not necessarily have impaired oxygenation functions at the onset of infection but may manifest rapid deterioration in oxygenation over time. Therefore, continual monitoring of oxygen saturation is recommended during oxygen therapy.

(2) Oxygen therapy as soon as possible.

Oxygen therapy is not necessary for patients whose oxygen saturation (SpO_2) is more than 93% or who have no obvious symptoms of respiratory distress without oxygen treatment. Oxygen therapy is strongly recommended to some severe patients with PaO_2/FiO_2 less than 300 mmHg but no obvious symptoms of respiratory distress.

(3) Treatment goal of oxygen therapy.

The treatment goal of oxygen therapy is to maintain the oxygen saturation (SpO_2) at 93%–96% for patients without chronic pulmonary disease and at 88%–92% for patients with chronic type II respiratory failure. Especially, the oxygen concentration should be increased to 92%–95% and $PaCO_2$ should be monitored for patients whose SpO_2 drops below 85% frequently during daily activities.

(4) Controlled oxygen therapy.

PaO_2/FiO_2 is a sensitive and accurate indicator of oxygenation function. The stability and monitorability of FiO_2 are very important for patients with disease progression and PaO_2/FiO_2 less than 300 mmHg. Controlled oxygen therapy is the first choice of treatment.

High-flow nasal cannula (HFNC) oxygen therapy is recommended for patients with the following conditions: $SpO_2<93\%$, $PaO_2/FiO_2<300$ mmHg, respiratory rate over 25 times per minute in a rest state, or remarkable progression on chest imaging. Patients should wear a surgical mask during HFNC treatment. The airflow of HFNC oxygen therapy should start at a low level and gradually increase up to 40–60 L/min when PaO_2/FiO_2 is between 200 and 300 mmHg and patients do not feel obvious chest tightness and shortness of breath. An initial flow of at least 60 L/min should be given immediately for patients with obvious respiratory distress.

Tracheal intubation is dependent on disease progression, systemic status and complications for patients with stable situation but with a low oxygenation index (<100 mmHg). Thus, a detailed evaluation of clinical conditions of the patients is very important before making a decision. Tracheal intubation should be performed as early as possible for patients with an oxygenation index less than 150 mmHg, worsening symptoms of respiratory distress or multiple organ dysfunction within 1–2 hours after high-flow (60 L/min) and high-concentration (>60%) HFNC oxygen therapy.

Older patients (>60 years old) with more complications or PaO_2/FiO_2 below 200 mmHg should be treated in ICU.

7.3.2 Mechanical Ventilation

(1) Noninvasive ventilation (NIV).

NIV is not strongly recommended for patients with COVID-19, who fail HFNC treatment. Some severe patients progress to acute respiratory distress syndrome rapidly. Excessive inflation pressure may cause gastric distension and intolerance which contributes to aspiration and worsens lung injury. A short-term (<2 hours) use of NIV can be closely monitored if the patient has acute left heart failure, chronic obstructive pulmonary disease or is immunosuppressed. Intubation should be performed as early as possible if improvement of respiratory distress symptoms or PaO_2/FiO_2 is not observed.

NIV with a double circuit is recommended. A virus filter should be installed between the mask and the exhalation valve when applying NIV with a single tube. Suitable masks should be chosen to reduce the risk of virus spread through air leakage.

(2) Invasive mechanical ventilation (IMV).

① Principles of IMV in critically ill patients. It is important to balance the ventilation and oxygenation demands and the risk of mechanical ventilation-related lung injury in the treatment of COVID-19.

● Strictly set the tidal volume at 4–8 mL/kg. In general, the lower the lung compliance is, the smaller the preset tidal volume should be.

● Maintain the platform pressure lower than 30 cmH_2O and driving pressure lower than 15 cmH_2O.

● Set positive end-expiratory pressure (PEEP) ventilation according to the ARDS's protocol.

● Ventilation frequency: 18–25 times per minute. Moderate hypercapnia is allowed.

● Administer sedative, analgesic, or muscle relaxant if the tidal volume, platform pressure and driving pressure are too high.

② Lung recruitment maneuvers. Lung recruitment maneuvers improve the heterogeneous distribution of lesions in patients with ARDS. However, it may result in severe respiratory and circulatory complications and therefore, the lung recruitment maneuvers are not routinely recommended. The assessment of lung expandability should be performed prior to the application.

(3) Prone position ventilation.

Most critically ill patients with COVID-19 respond well to prone ventilation, with a rapid improvement on oxygenation and lung mechanics. Prone ventilation is recommended as a routine strategy for patients with PaO_2/FiO_2 lower than 150 mmHg or with obvious imaging manifestations but no contraindications. Time course recommended for prone ventilation is more than 16 hours each time. The prone ventilation can be ceased once PaO_2/FiO_2 is higher than 150 mmHg for more than 4 hours in the supine position.

Prone ventilation while awake may be attempted for patients who have not been intubated or have no obvious respiratory distress, but with impaired oxygenation, or have consolidation in gravity-dependent lung zones on lung images. Procedures for at least 4 hours each time is recommended. Prone position can be performed several times per day depending on the effects and tolerance.

(4) Prevention of regurgitation and aspiration.

Gastric residual volume and gastrointestinal function should be routinely evaluated. Appropriate enteral nutrition is recommended to be given as early as possible. Nasointestinal feeding and continuous nasogastric decompression are recommended. Enteral nutrition should be suspended and aspiration with a 50 mL syringe should be done before transfer. If no contraindication exists, a 30° semi-sitting position is recommended.

(5) Fluid management.

Excessive fluid burden worsens hypoxemia for patients with COVID-19. To reduce pulmonary exudation and improve oxygenation, the amount of fluid should be strictly controlled while the patients' perfusion is ensured.

(6) Strategies to prevent ventilator-associated pneumonia (VAP) .

① Select an appropriate type of endotracheal tube.

② Use an endotracheal tube with subglottic suction (once every 2 hours, aspirated with a 20 mL empty syringe each time).

③ Place the endotracheal tube at the right position and correct depth, fix it properly and avoid pulling.

④ Maintain the airbag pressure at 30–35 cmH_2O and monitor it every 4 hours.

⑤ Monitor the airbag pressure and deal with water condensates when the position changes (two people cooperate to dump and pour the water condensates into a capped container with a pre-made chlorine-containing disinfectant), and deal with secretions accumulated in the airbag.

⑥ Clean up secretions from the mouth and the nose in time.

(7) Weaning of ventilation.

Sedatives are reduced and discontinued before awakening when the patients' PaO_2/FiO_2 is higher than 150 mmHg. Extubation should be performed as early as possible if possible. HFNC or NIV is used for sequential respiratory support after extubation.

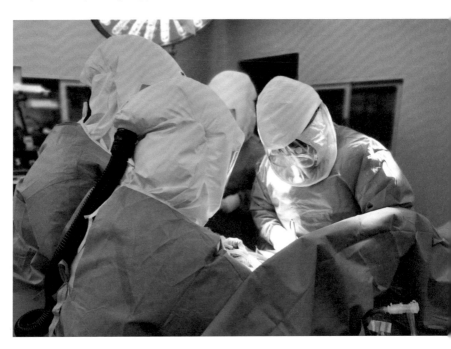

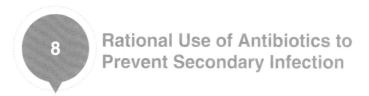

Rational Use of Antibiotics to Prevent Secondary Infection

COVID-19 is a disease of viral infection, therefore antibiotics are not recommended to prevent bacterial infection in mild or moderate patients; it should be used carefully in severe patients based on their conditions. Antibiotics can be used with discretion in patients who have the following conditions: extensive lung lesions, excess bronchial secretions, chronic airway diseases with a history of pathogen colonization in the lower respiratory tract, taking glucocorticoids at a dosage of ≥20 mg×7 d (in terms of prednisone). The options of antibiotics include quinolones, the second or third generation cephalothins, β-lactamase inhibitor compounds, etc. The antibiotics should be used for the prevention of bacterial infection in critically ill patients, especially those with invasive mechanical ventilation. The antibiotics such as carbapenems, β-lactamase inhibitor compounds, linezolid and vancomycin can be used in critically ill patients according to the individual risk factors.

The patients' symptoms, signs and indicators such as blood routine, C-reactive protein and procalcitonin need to be closely monitored during the treatment. When the change of a patient's condition is detected, a comprehensive clinical judgment needs to be made. When the secondary infection cannot be ruled out, qualified specimens need to be collected for testing by smear preparation, cultivation, nucleic acid, antigen and antibody, in order to determine the infectious agent as early as possible. Antibiotics can be empirically used under the following conditions: ① more expectoration, darker sputum color, especially yellow pus sputum; ② the rise of body temperature but not due to exacerbation of the underlying disease; ③ the marked increase of white blood cells and/or neutrophils; ④ with procalcitonin no less than 0.5 ng/mL; ⑤ exacerbation of oxygenation index or circulatory disturbance that is not caused by the viral infection; and the other conditions suspiciously caused by bacteria infections.

Some patients with COVID-19 are at the risk of secondary fungal infections due to weakened cellular immunity caused by viral infections, the use of glucocorticoid and/or broad-spectrum antibiotics. It is necessary to do microbiological detections for respiratory secretions such as smear preparation and cultivation for critically ill patients, and provide timely D-Glucose (G-test) and galactomannan (GM-test) of blood or bronchoalveolar lavage fluid for suspected patients.

It is necessary to be vigilant with possible invasive candidiasis infection. Anti-fungal therapy such as fluconazole or echinocandin is considered to be used under the following conditions: ① Patients are given broad-spectrum antibiotics for 7 days or more; ② Patients are treated with parenteral nutrition; ③ Patients have invasive examination or treatment; ④ Candida culture is tested positive in the specimens obtained from two body parts or more; ⑤ The level of D-Glucose increases significantly as a result of G-test.

It is necessary to be vigilant with possible invasive pulmonary aspergillosis. Anti-fungal therapy such as voriconazole, posaconazole, or echinocandin is considered to be used under the following conditions: ① Patients are given glucocorticoid for 7 days or more; ② Patients have agranulocytosis; ③ Patients have chronic obstructive pulmonary disease, and aspergillus culture is tested positive in the specimen obtained from the airway; ④ The level of galactomannan increases significantly as a result of GM-test.

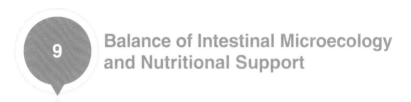

9 Balance of Intestinal Microecology and Nutritional Support

Some patients with COVID-19 have gastrointestinal symptoms (such as abdominal pain and diarrhea) due to direct viral infection of the intestinal mucosa or antiviral and anti-infective drugs. It is reported that the intestinal microecological balance is broken for patients with COVID-19, manifesting a significant reduction of the intestinal probiotics such as lactobacillus and bifidobacterium. Intestinal microecological imbalance may lead to bacterial translocation and secondary infection, so it is important to maintain the balance of intestinal microecology by microecological modulator and nutritional support.

9.1 Microecologics Intervention

(1) Microecologics can reduce bacterial translocation and secondary infection. It can increase dominant gut bacteria, inhibit harmful intestinal bacteria, reduce toxin production and infection caused by gut microflora dysbiosis.

(2) Microecologics can improve patients' gastrointestinal symptoms. It can reduce water in feces, improve fecal character and lower the frequency, and reduce diarrhea by inhibiting intestinal mucosal atrophy.

(3) The hospital can perform intestinal flora analysis if possible. Therefore, the intestinal flora disturbance can be discovered early according to the results. Antibiotics can be adjusted timely and probiotics can be prescribed, which can reduce the chances of intestinal bacterial translocation and gut-derived infection.

(4) Nutritional support is an important means to maintain intestinal microecological balance. Intestinal nutritional support should be applied timely on the basis of effective evaluations of nutritional risks,

gastrointestinal functions, and aspiration risks.

9.2 Nutritional Support

The severe and critically ill patients with COVID-19 are at high risks of malnutrition when they are under severe stress. Early evaluations of nutrition, gastrointestinal functions and aspiration risks, and timely enteral nutritional support are important to patients' prognoses.

(1) Oral feeding as the first choice: The early intestinal nutrition can provide nutritional support, nourish intestines, improve intestinal mucosal barrier and intestinal immunity, and maintain intestinal microecology.

(2) Enteral nutrition pathway: Severe and critically ill patients often harbor acute gastrointestinal damages, manifested as abdominal distension, diarrhea, and gastroparesis. For patients with tracheal intubation, intestinal nutrition tube indwelling is recommended for post-pyloric feeding.

(3) Selection of nutrient solution: For patients with intestinal damage, predigested short peptide preparations which are easy for intestinal absorption and utilization are recommended. For patients with good intestinal functions, whole-protein preparations with relatively high calories can be selected. For patients with hyperglycemia, nutritional preparations which are beneficial to glycemic controlling are recommended.

(4) Energy supply: According to the standard of 25 to 30 kcal/kg body weight, the target protein content is 1.2 to 2.0 g/kg daily.

(5) Means of nutrition supply: Pump infusion of nutrients can be used at a uniform speed, starting with a low dosage and gradually increasing. If possible, the nutrients can be heated before feeding to reduce intolerance.

(6) Parenteral nutritional support: The elderly patients who are at high aspiration risks or patients with apparent abdominal distension can be supported by parenteral nutrition temporarily, which can be gradually replaced by independent diet or enteral nutrition if their condition improves.

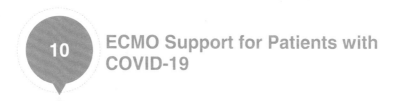

ECMO Support for Patients with COVID-19

COVID-19 is a novel, highly infectious disease primarily targeting pulmonary alveoli, which primarily damages the lungs of critically ill patients and leads to severe respiratory failure. For the application of extracorporeal membrane oxygenation (ECMO), medical professionals need to pay close attention to the follows: the time and means of intervention, anticoagulant and bleeding, coordination with mechanical ventilation, awake ECMO and the early rehabilitation training, weaning strategy, handling for complications, etc.

10.1 ECMO Intervention Timing

10.1.1 Salvage ECMO

In the state of mechanical ventilation support, measures such as lung protective ventilation strategy and prone position ventilation should be taken within 72 hours. At the onset of one of the following conditions, salvage ECMO intervention needs to be considered.

(1) $PaO_2/FiO_2 < 80$ mmHg (regardless of what the PEEP level is).

(2) Pplat≤30 mmHg, $PaCO_2 > 55$ mmHg.

(3) The onset of pneumothorax, air leakage>1/3 tidal volume, duration>48 h.

(4) Circulation deterioration, the dosage of norepinephrine>1 µg/(kg · min).

(5) Extracorporeal cardiopulmonary resuscitation (ECPR).

10.1.2 Replacement of ECMO

When the patient is not suitable for long-term mechanical ventilation support, i.e., the patient is not able to obtain the expected results, replacement of ECMO needs to be adopted immediately. At the onset of one of the following conditions, replacement of ECMO needs to be considered.

(1) Lung compliance decreases. After the pulmonary recruitment maneuvers, the compliance of the respiratory system is less than 10 mL/cmH$_2$O.

(2) Mediastinal emphysema or subcutaneous emphysema is exacerbated, and it is estimated that the parameters of mechanical ventilation support cannot be reduced within 48 hours.

(3) PaO$_2$/FiO$_2$ is lower than 100 mmHg, which cannot be improved by routine methods in 72 hours.

10.1.3 Early Awake ECMO

Early awake ECMO can be applied to patients who have been supported by mechanical ventilation with expected high parameters for more than 7 days, meet the necessary conditions of awake ECMO and might benefit from it. All the following conditions must be met.

(1) The patient is in a clear state of consciousness and is fully compliant. He or she understands how ECMO works and its maintenance requirements.

(2) The patient is not complicated with neuromuscular diseases.

(3) Pulmonary damage score: Murry>2.5.

(4) The patient has few pulmonary secretions. The time interval between the two airway suction procedures: more than 4 hours.

(5) The patient has stable hemodynamics and don't need assistance of vasoactive agents.

10.2 Cathetering Methods

As the ECMO supporting time is more than 7 days for most patients with COVID-19, the seldinger method should be adopted as much as possible for the ultrasound guided peripheral catheter insertion, which lowers the bleeding damages and infection risks along with intravascular cathterization, especially for the early awake ECMO patients. Intravascular catheterization may be considered only for the patients with poor blood vessel conditions, and whose catheterization cannot be identified and selected by ultrasound, or the patients for whom the seldinger method failed.

10.3 Mode Selection

(1) The first choice for patients with respiratory impairment is the V-V mode. The V-A mode should not be the first option just because of the possible circulation problems.

(2) For patients with respiratory failure, complicated with cardiac impairment, $PaO_2/FiO_2<100$ mmHg, the V-A-V mode ought to be selected with the total flux>6 L/min and V/A=0.5/0.5 is maintained by current limiting.

(3) For the COVID-19 patients without severe respiratory failure but complicated with serious cardiovascular outcomes leading to cardiogenic shock, the V-A mode ECMO ought to be selected. However, invasive positive pressure ventilation (IPPV) support is still needed and the awake ECMO should be avoided.

10.4 Flux Set-Value and Target Oxygen Supply

(1) The initial flux>80% cardiac output (CO) with a self-cycling rate<30%.

(2) $SpO_2>90\%$ should be maintained. $FiO_2<0.5$ is supported by mechanical ventilation or the other oxygen therapy.

(3) To ensure the target flux, 22 Fr vein access cannula is the first choice for the patients with a body weight below 80 kg, while 24 Fr is the first choice for those more than or equal to 80 kg.

10.5 Ventilation Setting

Normal ventilation maintenance is achieved by adjusting the level of sweep gas.

(1) The initial air flow is set as follows: blood flow : gas flow =1 : 1. The basic target is to maintain $PaCO_2$ lower than or equal to 45 mmHg. For the patients complicated with COPD, $PaCO_2$ is less than 80% of the basal level.

(2) The patients' spontaneous respiratory strength and respiratory frequency should be maintained at 10–20 breaths per minute without chief complaint of breathing difficulty from the patients.

(3) The sweep gas of the V-A mode needs to be set to ensure the value of the bloodstream out of the oxygenator membrane is 7.35–7.45 pH.

10.6 Anti-coagulation and Bleeding Prevention

(1) For the patients with no active bleeding, no visceral bleeding, and platelet count over 50×10^9/L, the recommended initial heparin dosage is 50 IU/kg. For the patients complicated with bleeding or platelet count less than 50×10^9/L, the recommended initial heparin dosage is 25 IU/kg.

(2) The activated partial thromboplastin time (APTT) being 40–60 seconds is proposed to be the target of anticoagulation maintenance dosage. The trend of D-dimer change should be taken into consideration at the same time.

(3) Heparin-free operation may be performed in the following circumstances: The ECMO support must continue but there is fatal bleeding or active bleeding that has to be controlled, with the whole heparin coated loop, catheterization, blood flow over 3 L/min. The recommend operation period is less than 24 hours and the replacing devices and consumables need to be prepared.

(4) Heparin resistance: Under some conditions of adopting heparin, when APTT is not able to reach the standard and blood coagulation happens, the activity of plasma antithrombin Ⅲ (AT Ⅲ) needs to be monitored. If the activity reduces, fresh frozen plasma needs to be supplemented to restore its sensitivity to heparin.

(5) Heparin induced thrombopenia (HIT): When HIT happens, we recommend to perform plasma exchange therapy, or to replace heparin with argatroban.

10.7 Weaning from ECMO and Mechanical Ventilation

(1) If a patient treated by V-V ECMO combined with mechanical ventilation satisfies the awake ECMO condition, we suggest to first try to remove the artificial airway, unless the patient has ECMO related complications, or the expected time of removal of all the assisting machines is less than 48 hours.

(2) For a patient who has too much airway secretions that frequent artificial suction clearance is needed, who is expected to have a long-term mechanical ventilation support, whose PaO$_2$/FiO$_2$ is over 150 mmHg for more than 48 hours, whose lung image changes for the better, and whose damages related to mechanical ventilation pressure have been controlled, the ECMO assistance may be removed. The ECMO intubation is not recommended to keep.

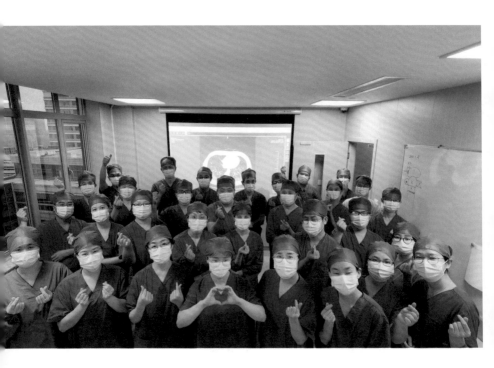

11 Convalescent Plasma Therapy for Patients with COVID-19

Since Behring and Kitasato reported the therapeutic effects of diphtheria antitoxin plasma in 1891, plasma therapy had become an important means of pathogen immunotherapy for acute infectious diseases. The disease progression is rapid for severe and critically ill patients with an emerging infectious disease. In the early phase, the pathogens damage the target organs directly and then lead to severe immuno-pathological damage. The passive immune antibodies can effectively and directly neutralize the pathogens, which reduces the damage of the target organs and then blocks the subsequent immune-pathological damages. During multiple global epidemic outbreaks, WHO also emphasized that "convalescent plasma therapy is one of the most recommended potential therapies, and it had been used during other epidemic outbreaks". Since the outbreak of COVID-19, the initial mortality rate has been rather high due to the lack of specific and effective treatments. As mortality rate is an important metric that the public concerns about, clinic treatments which can lower the fatality rate of critical cases effectively are key to avoiding public panic. As a provincial-level hospital in Zhejiang province, FAHZU is responsible to receive and treat patients from Hangzhou and the critically ill ones all over Zhejiang province. There are abundant potential convalescent plasma donors prepared in FAHZU, whose plasma could be applied to be infused for critically ill patients in need of convalescent plasma treatment.

11.1 Plasma Collection

In addition to the common requirements of blood donation and procedures, the following details should be noted.

11.1.1 Donors

At least 2 weeks after recovery and discharge (the result of the nucleic acid test of the sample taken from the lower respiratory tract remains negative for over 14 days). The age is between 18 and 55. The body weight is over 50 kg for male and over 45 kg for female. It has been at least 1 week since last glucocorticoid usage and more than 2 weeks since last blood donation.

11.1.2 Collection Method

Plasmapheresis, 200–400 mL each time (based on medical consultation).

11.1.3 Post-collection Testing

In addition to the general quality test and the test of blood-borne disease, the blood samples need to be tested for the following.

(1) The nucleic acid test for SARS-CoV-2.

(2) A qualitative test of SARS-CoV-2 specific IgG and IgM detection with 160-fold dilution; a qualitative test of whole antibody detection with 320-fold dilution. If possible, keep more than 3 mL plasma for viral neutralization experiments.

Comparing virus neutralization titer and luminescent IgG antibody quantitative detection, we have found that the present detection of specific IgG antibody for SARS-CoV-2 does not fully demonstrate the actual virus neutralization capability of the plasma. Therefore, we suggested the virus neutralization test as the first choice, or the test of overall antibody level with 320-fold dilution of the plasma.

11.2 Clinical Use of the Convalescent Plasma

11.2.1 Indications

(1) Severe or critically ill patients with COVID-19 tested positive for the virus in the respiratory tract.

(2) Patients with COVID-19 who are not severe or critically ill, but in a state of immunity suppression; or who have low CT values in the virus nucleic acid testing but with a rapid disease progression in the lungs.

Note: In principle, the convalescent plasma should not be used on COVID-19 patients with an over-3-week disease course. However, in clinical practice, we have found that the convalescent plasma therapy is effective for patients with a disease course exceeding 3 weeks and whose virus nucleic acid tests continuously show positive results with respiratory tracts specimen. It can speed up virus clearance, increase the numbers of the plasma lymphocytes and natural killer (NK) cells, reduce the level of plasma lactic acid, and improve renal functions.

11.2.2 Contraindications

(1) Patients have an allergy history of plasma, sodium citrate and methylene blue.

(2) For patients with history of autoimmune system diseases or selective IgA deficiency, the application of convalescent plasma should be evaluated cautiously by doctors.

11.2.3 Infusion Plan

In general, the dosage of convalescent plasma therapy is more than or equal to 400 mL for one infusion, or no less than 200 mL per infusion for multiple infusions.

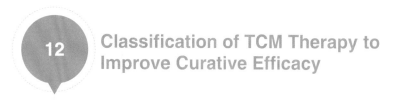

Classification of TCM Therapy to Improve Curative Efficacy

12. 1 Classification and Stages

According to its development, COVID-19 can be divided into 4 stages: early, middle, critical and recovery stage. At the early stage, the disease has two main types, "wet lungs" and "external cold and internal heat". The middle stage is characterized by "intermittent cold and heat". The critical stage is characterized by "internal block of epidemic toxin". The recovery stage is characterized by "qi deficiency of the lung and the spleen". The disease initially belongs to wet lung syndrome. Due to fever, both intermittent cold and heat treatments are recommended. In the middle stage, cold, dampness, and heat coexist, belonging to "cold-heat mixture" in terms of traditional Chinese medicine (TCM). Both cold and heat therapies should be taken into consideration. According to the theory of TCM, heat should be treated with cold drugs. But cold drugs impair Yang and lead to a cold spleen and stomach and cold-heat mixture in the middle-Jiao. Therefore, in this stage both cold and heat therapies should be taken into consideration. Because cold-heat symptoms are commonly seen in patients with COVID-19, the cold-heat therapy is better than other approaches.

12.2 Classification-Based Therapy

(1) Cold-damp and stagnating lung
    Chinese Ephedra 6 g
    Apricot Kernel 10 g
    Coix Seed 30 g
    Liquoric Root 6 g
    Baical Skullcap Root 15 g

Wrinkled Giant Hyssop 10 g
Common Reed Rhizome 30 g
Basket Fern 15 g
Indian Bread 20 g
Atractylodes Rhizome 12 g
Officinal Magnolia Bark 12 g

(2) External cold and internal heat
Chinese Ephedra 9 g
Unprepared Gypsum 30 g
Apricot Kernel 10 g
Liquoric Root 6 g
Baical Skullcap Root 15 g
Trichosanthes Peel 20 g
Bitter Orange 15 g
Officinal Magnolia Bark 12 g
Tripterospermum Cordifolium 20 g
Mulberry Root-Bark 15 g
Pinellia Tuber 12 g
Indian Bread 20 g
Platycodon Root 9 g

(3) Intermittent cold and heat
Pinellia Tuber 12 g
Baical Skullcap Root 15 g
Coftis Root 6 g
Dried Ginger 6 g
Chinese Date 15 g
Kudzuvine Root 30 g
Costustoot 10 g
Indian Bread 20 g
Thunberg Fritillary Bulb 15 g
Coix Seed 30 g
Liquoric Root 6 g

(4) Internal block of epidemic toxin
  Oral administration of cheongsimhwan for treatment.

(5) Qi deficiency of the lung and the spleen
  Membranous Milkvetch Root 30 g
  Pilose Asiabell Root 20 g
  Parched White Atractylodes Rhizome 15 g
  Indian Bread 20 g
  Amomum Fruit 6 g
  Polygonatum Falcatum Rhizome 15 g
  Pinellia Tuber 10 g
  Tangerine Peel 6 g
  Chinese Yam Rhizome Batatatis 20 g
  Hindu Lotus Seed 15 g
  Chinese Date 15 g

Patients in different stages should be treated by different approaches. Boil the herbs in water twice and take a dose per day with half in the morning and half in the evening.

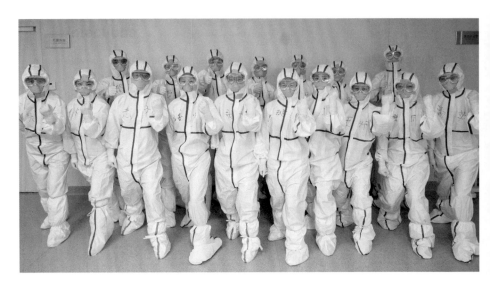

13 Management of Drug Use for Patients with COVID-19

Patients with COVID-19 are often complicated with underlying diseases receiving multiple types of drugs. Therefore, we should pay more attention to adverse drug reactions and drug interactions so as to avoid drug-induced organ damage and improve the success rate of treatment.

13.1 Identification of Adverse Drug Reactions

It has been demonstrated that the incidence of abnormal liver function is 51.9% in patients with COVID-19 who have received lopinavir/ritonavir combined Arbidol antiviral treatment. Multivariate analysis revealed that antiviral agents and more concomitant medications are two independent risk factors of abnormal liver function. Therefore, monitoring of the adverse drug reactions should be strengthened and the unnecessary drug combinations should be reduced. The main adverse reactions of antiviral agents include the follows.

(1) Lopinavir/ritonavir and darunavir/cobicistat: diarrhea, nausea, vomit, an increase of serum aminotransferase, jaundice, dyslipidemia, an increase of lactic acid, etc. Symptoms will disappear after drug withdrawal.

(2) Arbidol: an increase of serum aminotransferase and jaundice. While combined with lopinavir, the incidence rate is even higher. The symptoms will disappear after drug withdrawal. Sometimes a slowdown of the heart rate could be induced, thus it is necessary to avoid the combination of Arbidol with β -receptor inhibitors such as metoprolol and propranolol. We suggest to stop taking the drugs when the heart

rate drops below 60/min.

(3) Favipiravir: elevation of plasma uric acid, diarrhea, neutropenia, shock, fulminant hepatitis, acute kidney injury, etc. The adverse reactions are commonly seen in elderly patients or patients complicated with cytokine storm.

(4) Chloroquine phosphate: dizziness, headache, nausea, vomit, diarrhea, different kinds of skin rash. The most severe adverse reaction is cardiac arrest, while the main adverse reaction is the ocular toxicity. An electrocardiogram needs to be examined before drug administration. The drug should be prohibited for patients with arrhythmia (e.g., conduction block), retinal disease, or hearing loss.

13.2 Monitoring of Plasma Concentration of Therapeutic Drugs

Some antiviral and antibacterial drugs need therapeutic drug monitoring (TDM). Table 2.1 presents the potential interaction of such drugs and their contraindications in combined medication. Upon the onset of aberrations of plasma concentration of therapeutic drugs, the treatment regimens need to be adjusted by considering clinical symptoms and concomitant drugs.

Table 2.1 The range of concentrations and points for attention of the common TDM drugs for the COVID-19 patients

Drug Name	Timing of Bood Collection	Range of Concentrations	Principle of Dosage Adjustment
Lopinavir/ ritonavir	(peak) Within 30 min after drug administration. (trough) Within 30 min before drug administration	Lopinavir: (trough)>1 µg/mL (peak)<8.2 µg/mL	Correlated with drug efficacy and side effects
Imipenem	Within 10 min before current drug administration	1–8 µg/mL	Interpreting plasma concentration of therapeutic drugs based on minimum inhibitory concentration (MIC) of the pathogen testing, and adjusting the therapeutic regimen
Meropenem	Within10 min before current drug administration	1–16 µg/mL	

(To be continued)

(Table 2.1)

Drug Name	Timing of Bood Collection	Range of Concentrations	Principle of Dosage Adjustment
Vancomycin	Within 30 min before current drug administration	10–20 mg/L (15–20 mg/L for the severe methicillin resistant staphylococcus aureus infection)	The trough concentration correlates with the failure rate of anti-infective therapy and renal toxicity. When the concentration is overly high, dosage frequency or single dose is required to be lowered
Linezolid	Within 30 min before the drug administration	2–7 μg/mL	The trough concentration correlates with myelosuppression adverse reactions. The blood routine test needs to be closely monitored
Voriconazole	Within 30 min before the drug administration	1–5.5 μg/mL	The trough concentration correlates with the therapeutic efficacy and adverse reactions such as impaired liver function

13.3 Paying attention to the potential drug interactions

Antiviral drugs such as lopinavir/ritonavir are metabolized through the enzyme CYP3A in the liver. When patients receive concomitant medications, the potential drug interactions need to be carefully screened. Table 2.2 shows interactions between antiviral drugs and common drugs for underlying diseases.

Table 2.2 Potential interactions and contraindications of some antiviral and antibacterial drugs

Drug Name	Potential Interactions	Contraindications in Combined Medication
Lopinavir/ ritonavir	When combined with drugs associated with CYP3A metabolism (e.g., statins, immune suppressors such as tacrolimus, voriconazole), the plasma concentration of the combined drug may increase, leading to 153%, 5.9–fold, 13–fold increase of the AUC of rivaroxaban, atrovastatin, midazolam, respectively. Pay attention to clinical symptoms and apply the TDM	Combined use with amiodarone (fatal arrhythmia), quetiapine(severe coma), simvastatin (rhabdomyolysis) is prohibited

(To be continued)

Part Two Diagnosis and Treatment

(Table 2.3)

Drug Name	Potential Interactions	Contraindications in Combined Medication
Darunavir/ cobicistat	When combined with drugs associated with CYP3A and/or CYP2D6 metabolism, the plasma concentration of the combined drugs may increase. See lopinavir/ritonavir for drugs that may cause potenitial interactions	See lopinavir/ritonavir
Arbidol	It interacts with CYP3A4, UGT1A9 substrates, inhibitors, and inducers	–
Favipiravir	① Theophyllinum increases the bioavailability of favipiravir. ② It increases the bioavailability of acetaminophen by 1.79 folds. ③ Its combination with pyrazinamide increases the plasma uric acid level. ③ Its combination with repaglinide increases the plasma repaglinide level	–
Chloroquine phosphate	–	Not to be administrated together with the drugs that may result in the prolonged Q-T interval (such as moxifloxacin, azithromycin, amiodarone, etc.)

Note: "–": no relevant data.
TDM: therapeutic drug monitoring.
AUC: area under the curve.
UGT1A9: uridine diphosphate glucosidase 1A9.

13.4 Avoiding Medical Damage in Special Populations

Special populations include pregnant women, patients with hepatic and renal insufficiency, patients supported by mechanical ventilation, patients under continuous renal replacement therapy (CRRT) or, extracorporeal membrane oxygenation (ECMO), etc. The following aspects need to be noted during drug administration.

(1) For pregnant women, lopinavir/ritonavir tablets could be administrated, but favipiravir and chloroquine phosphate are prohibited.

(2) For patients with hepatic insufficiency, drugs that are excreted unchanged through the kidney are preferred, such as penicillin and cephalosporins, etc.

(3) For patients with renal insufficiency (including those on hemodialysis), drugs that are metabolized through the liver or excreted

through double channels of the liver-kidney are preferred, such as linezolid, moxifloxacin, ceftriaxone, etc.

(4)For patients under CRRT for 24 hours, vancomycin can be administrated, and the recommended regimen is as follows: loading dose 1.0 g and maintenance dose 0.5 g, q12h. For imipenem, the maximum daily dosage should not exceed 2.0 g.

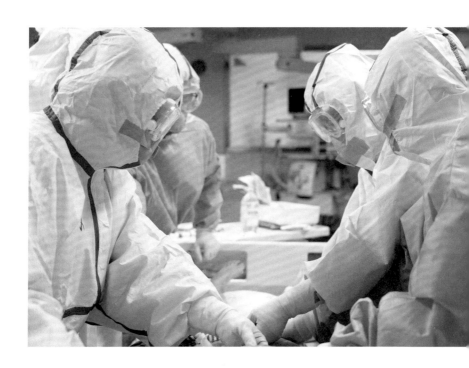

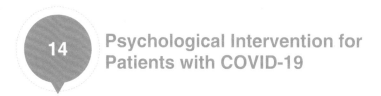

Psychological Intervention for Patients with COVID-19

14.1 Psychological Stress and Symptoms of Patients with COVID-19

Confirmed COVID-19 patients often have symptoms such as regret and resentment, loneliness and helplessness, depression, anxiety and phobia, irritation and sleep deprivation. Some patients may have panic attacks. Psychological evaluations in the isolated wards demonstrated that about 48% of confirmed patients with COVID-19 manifested psychological stress during early admission, most of which were from their emotional response to stress. The percentage of delirium is high among the critically ill patients. There is even a report of encephalitis induced by the SARS-CoV-2 leading to psychological symptoms such as unconsciousness and irritability.

14.2 Establishing a Dynamic Mechanism for Evaluation and Warning of Psychological Crisis

Patients' mental states (individual psychological stress, mood, sleep quality, and pressure) should be monitored every week after admission and before discharge. Self-rating tools include: Self-Reporting Questionnaire 20 (SRQ-20), Patient Health Questionnaire 9 (PHQ-9) and the Generalized Anxiety Disorder 7-Item (GAD-7) Scale. The peer-rating tools include: Hamilton Depression Rating Scale (HAMD), Hamilton Anxiety Rating Scale (HAMA), Positive and Negative Syndrome Scale (PANSS). In such a special environment as the isolated wards, we suggest that patients should be guided to complete the questionnaires through their cell phones. The doctors can interview and perform scale assessing through face-to-face or online discussion. More body languages are recommended for communication when doctors wear protective clothing.

14.3 Intervention and Treatment Based on the Assessment

14.3.1 Principles of Intervention and Treatment

Psychological intervention is suggested for mild patients. Psychological self-adjustment includes breathing relaxation training and mindfulness training. For moderate to severe patients, intervention and treatment by combining medication and psychotherapy are suggested. New antidepressants, anxiolytics, and benzodiazepines can be prescribed to improve the patients' mood and sleep quality. The second generation antipsychotics such as olanzapine and quetiapine can be used to improve psychotic symptoms such as illusion and delusion.

14.3.2 Recommendation of Psychotropic Medications in Elderly Patients

The medical conditions of middle-aged or elderly patients with COVID-19 are often complicated by physical diseases such as hypertension and diabetes. Therefore, when selecting psychotropic medications, the drug interactions and their effects on respiration must be fully considered. We recommend using citalopram, escitalopram, etc. to improve depression and anxiety symptoms; using benzodiazepines such as estazolam, alprazolam, etc. to improve anxiety and sleep quality; using olanzapine, quetiapine, etc. to improve psychotic symptoms.

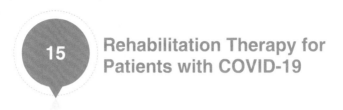

Rehabilitation Therapy for Patients with COVID-19

Severe and critically ill patients suffer from different degrees of dysfunction, especially respiratory insufficiency, dyskinesia and cognitive impairment, during both acute and recovery stages.

The goal of early rehabilitation intervention is to reduce breathing difficulties, relieve symptoms, ease anxiety and depression, and lower the incidence of complications. The process of early rehabilitation intervention is: rehabilitation assessment → therapy → reassessment.

15.1 Rehabilitation Assessment

Based on general clinical assessment, especially functional evaluation, including respiration, cardiac status, motion and ADL should be emphasized. Focus on respiratory rehabilitation assessment, which includes the evaluation of thoracic activity, diaphragm activity amplitude, respiratory pattern and frequency, etc.

15.2 Rehabilitation Therapy

The rehabilitation therapy of severe or critically ill patients with COVID-19 mainly includes position management, respiratory exercise, active cycle of breathing techniques, positive expiratory pressure trainer, and physical therapy.

15.2.1 Position Management

Postural drainage may reduce the influence of sputum on the respiratory tract, which is especially important to improve the patients' V/Q. Patients must learn to tip themselves into a position which allows gravity to assist in draining excretion from lung lobes or lung segments. For patients using sedatives and suffering from consciousness disturbance, a standing-up bed or the bed head elevation ($30° \rightarrow 45° \rightarrow 60°$) may be applied if the patient's condition permits. Standing is the best body position for the patient's breathing in a resting state, which can effectively increase the patient's respiratory efficiency and maintain lung volume. As long as the patient feels good, let the patient take a standing position and gradually keep standing longer and longer.

15.2.2 Respiratory Exercise

Exercise can fully expand the lungs, help the excretions from pulmonary alveoli and airway expel into the large airway so that sputum would not accumulate at the bottom of the lungs. It increases the vital capacity and enhances lung function. Deep-slow breathing and chest expansion breathing combined with shoulder expansion are the two major techniques of respiratory exercises.

(1) Deep-slow breathing. While inhaling, the patient should try his/her best to move the diaphragm actively. The breathing should be as deep and slow as possible to avoid the reduction of respiratory efficiency caused by fast-shallow breathing. Compared with thoracic breathing, this kind of breathing needs less muscle strength but has better tidal volume and V/Q value, which can be used to adjust breathing when shortness of breath happens.

(2) Chest expansion breathing combined with shoulder expansion. It can improve the pulmonary ventilation. When taking a deep-slow breath, one expands his/her chest and shoulders while inhaling, and moves back his/her chest and shoulders while exhaling. Due to the special pathological factors of viral pneumonia, suspending breathing for a long time should be avoided in order not to increase the burden of work of breathing, the heart, as well as oxygen consumption. Meanwhile, the patients should avoid moving too fast and it's best to adjust the respiratory rate to 12–15 breaths/min.

15.2.3 Active Cycle of Breathing Techniques

It can effectively remove bronchus excretion and improve lung function without exacerbation of hypoxemia and airflow obstruction. It consists of three stages (breathing control, thoracic expansion and exhalation). How to form a cycle of breathing should be developed according to the patient's condition.

15.2.4 Positive Expiratory Pressure Trainer

The pulmonary interstitium of patients with COVID-19 has been severely damaged. In mechanical ventilation, low pressure and low tidal volume are required to avoid damages to the pulmonary interstitium. Therefore, after the removal of mechanical ventilation, positive expiratory pressure trainer can be used to help the movement of excretions from the low-volume lung segments to the high-volume segments, lowering the difficulty of expectoration. Expiratory positive pressure can be generated through air flow vibration, which vibrates the airway to achieve airway supporting. The excretions can then be removed as the high-speed expiratory flow moves the excretions.

15.2.5 Physical Therapy

Physical therapy includes ultrashort wave, oscillators, external diaphragm pacemaker, electrical muscle stimulation, etc.

16 Lung Transplantation in Patients with COVID-19

Lung transplantation is an effective treatment approach for final-stage chronic lung diseases. However, it is rarely reported that lung transplantation has been performed to treat acute infectious lung diseases. Based on current clinical practice and results, FAHZU summarized this chapter as a reference for medical workers. In general, following the principles of exploration, doing the best to save life, highly selective and high protection, if lung lesions are not significantly improved after adequate and reasonable medical treatment, and the patient is in critical condition, lung transplantation could be considered with other evaluations.

16.1 Pre-transplantation Assessment

16.1.1 Age

It is recommended that the recipients are not older than 70 years old. Patients over 70 years old are subject to careful evaluation of other organ functions and postoperative recovery capability.

16.1.2 Course of the Disease

There is no direct correlation between the length of the disease course and the severity of the disease. However, for patients with short disease courses (shorter than 4–6 weeks), a full medical assessment is recommended to evaluate whether adequate medication, ventilator assistance, and ECMO support have been provided.

16.1.3 Pulmonary Status

Based on the parameters collected from lung CT, ventilator, and ECMO, it is necessary to evaluate whether there is any chance of recovery.

16.1.4 Functional Assessment of Other Major Organs

Evaluation of the consciousness status of patients in critical condition using brain CT scan and electroencephalography is crucial, as most of them would have been sedated for an extended period. Cardiac assessments, including electrocardiogram and echocardiography that focus on size of the right heart, pulmonary artery pressure and function of the left heart, are highly recommended. The levels of serum creatinine and bilirubin should also be monitored. Patients with liver failure and renal failure should not be subjected to lung transplantation until the functions of the liver and kidney are recovered.

16.1.5 The Nucleic Acid Test of COVID-19

The patient should be tested negative for at least two consecutive nucleic acid tests at a sampling interval beyond 24 hours. Given the increased incidents of COVID-19 test result returning from negative to positive after treatment, it is recommended to revise the standard to three consecutive negative results. Ideally, negative results should be observed in all body fluid samples, including blood, sputum, nasopharynx, broncho-alveolar lavage, urine, and feces. Considering the difficulty in operation, at least the testing of sputum and broncho-alveolar lavage samples should be negative.

16.1.6 Assessment of Infection Status

With the extended in-patient treatment, some patients with COVID-19 may have multiple bacterial infections, and thus a full medical assessment is recommended to evaluate the situation of infection control, especially for multidrug-resistant bacterial infection. Moreover, post-procedure antibacterial treatment plans should be formed to estimate the risk of post-procedure infections.

16.1.7 Preoperative Assessment Procedures for Lung Transplantation in Patients with COVID-19

A treatment plan proposed by the ICU team → Multidisciplinary therapy → Comprehensive medical examination → Analyses and treatment of relative contraindications → Pre-habilitation before lung transplantation.

16.2 Contraindications

Please refer to A Consensus Document for the Selection of Lung Transplant Candidates: 2014–An Update from the Pulmonary Transplantation Council of the International Society for Heart and Lung Transplantation Issued by the International Society for Heart and Lung Transplantation (updated in 2014).

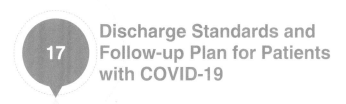

Discharge Standards and Follow-up Plan for Patients with COVID-19

17

17.1 Discharge Standards

(1) Body temperature remains normal for at least 3 days (ear temperature is lower than 37.5 ℃).

(2) Respiratory symptoms are significantly improved.

(3)The nucleic acid is tested negative for respiratory tract pathogen twice consecutively (at a sampling interval beyond 24 hours); the nucleic acid test of stool samples can be performed at the same time if possible.

(4) Lung imaging shows obvious improvement in lesions.

(5)There are no complications or comorbidities which require hospitalization.

(6) The patients should achieve a blood oxygen saturation (SpO_2) level of over 93% without assisted oxygen inhalation.

(7) Discharge is approved by multi-disciplinary medical team.

17.2 Medication after Discharge

Generally, antiviral drugs are not necessary after discharge. Treatments for symptoms can be applied if patients have a mild cough, a poor appetite, thick tongue coating, etc. Antiviral drugs can be used after discharge for patients with multiple lung lesions in the first 3 days after their nucleic acid are tested negative.

17.3 Home Isolation

Patients must continue with two weeks of isolation after discharge. Recommended home isolation conditions include the follows.

(1) Independent living area with frequent ventilation and disinfection.

(2) Avoid contacting with infants, the elderly and people with weak immune functions at home.

(3) Patients and their family members must wear a mask, and wash hands frequently.

(4) Body temperature should be taken twice a day (in the morning and evening) . Pay close attention to any changes in the patients' condition.

17.4 Follow-up

A specialized doctor should be arranged for each discharged patient's follow-ups. The first follow-up call should be made within 48 hours after discharge. The outpatient follow-up will be carried out 1 week, 2 weeks, and 1 month after discharge. Examinations include liver and kidney functions, blood test, nucleic acid test of sputum and stool samples, and pulmonary function test or lung CT scan should be reviewed according to the patient's condition. Follow-up phone calls should be made 3 and 6 months after discharge.

17.5 Management of Patients Tested Positive Again after Discharge

Strict discharge standards have been implemented in FAHZU. There is no discharged case in FAHZU whose sputum and stool samples are tested positive again in the follow-ups. However, there are some reported cases that patients are tested positive again after being discharged based on the standards of national guidelines (negative results from at least 2 consecutive throat swabs collected at an interval of 24 hours; body temperature remaining normal for 3 days, symptoms significantly improved; obvious absorption of inflammation on lung images). It is mainly due to sample collection errors and false negative testing results. For these patients, the following strategies are recommended.

(1) Isolation according to the standards for patients with COVID-19.

(2) Continuing to provide antiviral treatment which has been proved to

be effective during prior hospitalization.

(3) Discharge only when improvement is observed on lung imaging and the sputum and stool are tested negative for 3 consecutive times (at an interval of 24 hours).

(4) Home isolation and follow-up visits after discharge in accordance with the requirements mentioned above.

Part Three

Nursing

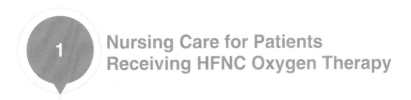

1 Nursing Care for Patients Receiving HFNC Oxygen Therapy

1.1 Assessing

Provide detailed information of the High-Flow Nasal Cannula(HFNC) oxygen therapy to get the patient's cooperation before implementation. Use low dose sedative with close monitoring if necessary. Choose a proper nasal catheter based on the diameter of the patient's nasal cavity. Adjust the head strap tightness and use decompression plaster to prevent device-related pressure injuries on the facial skin. Maintain the water level in the humidifier chamber. Titrate the flow rate, the fraction of inspired oxygen (FiO_2), and the water temperature based on the patient's respiratory demands and tolerance.

1.2 Monitoring

Report to the attending physician to seek medical decision of replacing HFNC by mechanical ventilation if any of the followings occur: hemodynamic instability, respiratory distress evidenced by obvious contraction of accessory muscles, hypoxemia persists despite oxygen therapy, deterioration of consciousness, the respiratory rate over 40 breaths/min continuously, and a significant amount of sputum.

1.3 Treatment of Secretions

Patients' drool, snot, and sputum should be wiped with tissue paper and disposed in a sealed container with chlorine-containing disinfectant (2500 mg/L). Alternatively, secretions can be removed by oral mucus extractor or suctioning tube and be disposed in a sputum collector with chlorine-containing disinfectant (2500 mg/L).

2 Nursing Care for Patients with Mechanical Ventilation

2.1 Intubation Procedures

The number of the medical staff should be limited to the minimum number that can ensure the patients' safety. Medical staff should wear powered air-purifying respirator as PPE. Before intubation, perform administration of sufficient analgesia and sedative, use muscle relaxant if necessary, and closely monitor the hemodynamic response during intubation. Within 30 minutes after completion of intubation, staff should reduce movement in the ward, continuously purify and disinfect the room by a plasma air disinfector.

2.2 Analgesia, Sedation and Delirium Management

Set a target of analgesia and sedation every day. Assess pain by Critical-Care Pain Observation Tool (CPOT) every 4 hours, measure sedation by Richmond Agitation-Sedation Scale (RASS) or by Bispectral Index (BIS) every 2 hours. Titrate the infusion rate of analgesics and sedatives to achieve the target. For the known painful procedures, preemptive analgesia is administered. Perform CAM-ICU delirium screening in every shift to ensure an early diagnosis for patients with COVID-19. Apply centralization strategy for delirium prevention, including pain relief, sedation, communication, quality sleep, and early mobilization.

2.3 Prevention of Ventilator-Associated Pneumonia (VAP)

The ventilator bundle is used to reduce VAP, which includes hand washing; raising the tilt angle of the patient's bed by 30°–45°. If no contradiction is presented, perform oral care every 4 to 6 hours by using a disposable oral mucus extractor; maintain endotracheal tube (ETT) cuff pressure at 30–35 cmH$_2$O every 4 hours; provide enteral nutritional support and monitor gastric residual volume every 4 hours; daily evaluate for ventilator removal; using washable tracheal tubes for continuous subglottic suctioning combined with 10 mL syringe suctioning every 1 to 2 hours, and adjusting the suctioning frequency according to the actual amount of secretions. Dispose retentate below the glottis: The syringe containing the subglottic secretions is immediately used to aspirate an appropriate amount of chlorine-containing disinfectant (2500 mg/L), and then is re-capped and disposed of in a sharp container.

2.4 Sputum Suction

(1) Suctioning. Use a closed sputum suction system, including closed suction catheter and closed disposable collection bag, to reduce the formation of aerosol and droplets.
(2) Collection of sputum specimen. Use a closed suction catheter and a matching collection bag to reduce exposure to droplets.

2.5 Disposal of Condensation from Ventilators

Use disposable ventilator tubing with dual-loop heating wire and automatic humidifier to reduce the formation of condensation. Two nurses cooperate to dump the condensation promptly into a capped container with chlorine-containing disinfectant (2500 mg/L). The container can then be directly put in a washing machine, which can be heated up to 90℃, for automatic cleaning and disinfection.

2.6 Nursing Care for the Prone Position Ventilation (PPV)

Before changing the position, secure the position of tubing and check all the joints to reduce the risk of disconnection. Change the patient's position every 2 hours .

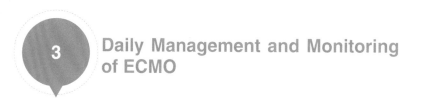

Daily Management and Monitoring of ECMO

3

(1) Extracorporeal membrane oxygenation (ECMO) equipment should be managed by ECMO perfusionists, and the following items should be checked and recorded every hour: pump flow rate/rotation speed; blood flow; oxygen flow; oxygen concentration; ensuring that the temperature controller is flowing; temperature setting and actual temperature; preventing clots in circuit; no pressure to the cannulae and the circuit tubing is not kinked, or no " shaking" of ECMO tubes; patient's urine color with special attention to red or dark brown urine; pre & post membrane pressure as required by the doctor.

(2) The following items during every shift should be monitored and recorded: Check the depth and fixation of cannula to ensure that the ECMO circuit interfaces are firm; check the water level line of the temperature controller, the power supply of the machine and the connection of the oxygen, the cannula site for any bleeding and swelling; measure leg circumference and observe whether the lower limb on the operation side is swollen; observe lower limbs, such as dorsalis pedis artery pulse, skin temperature, color, etc.

(3) Daily monitor post membrane blood gas analysis.

(4)The basic goal of ECMO anticoagulation management is to achieve a moderate anticoagulation effect, which ensures that certain coagulation activity under the premise of avoiding excessive activation of coagulation. That is to maintain the balance among anticoagulation, coagulation and fibrinolysis. The patients should be injected with heparin sodium (25–50 IU/kg) at the time of intubation and maintained with heparin sodium (7.5–20 IU/kg/h) during the pump flow period. The dosage of heparin sodium should be adjusted according to

APTT results which should be held between 40–60 seconds. During the anticoagulation period, the number of skin punctures should be reduced as less as possible, and operations should be taken gently. The status of bleeding should also be observed carefully.

(5) Implement the "ultra-protective lung ventilation" strategy to avoid or reduce the occurrence of ventilator-related lung injury. It is recommended that the initial tidal volume is less than 6 mL/kg and the intensity of spontaneous breathing is retained (Breathing frequency should be between 10 and 20 breaths/min).

(6) Closely observe the vital signs of patients, maintain MAP between 60 and 65 mmHg, with CVP less than 8 mmHg, SpO_2 over 90%, and monitor the status of urine volume and blood electrolytes.

(7) Transfuse through the post membrane, avoiding infusion of fat emulsion and propofol.

(8) Based on the monitoring records, evaluate the ECMO oxygenator function during each shift.

4 Nursing Care of ALSS

Nursing care of artificial liver support system (ALSS) is mainly divided into two kinds: nursing care during treatment and intermittent care. Nursing staff should closely observe the conditions of patients, standardize the operating procedures, focus on key points and deal with complications timely in order to successfully complete ALSS treatment.

4.1 Nursing Care During Treatment

It refers to nursing during each stage of ALSS treatment. The overall operation process can be summarized as follows: operators' own preparation, patients' evaluation, installation, pre-flushing, running, parameter adjustment, weaning and recording. The following are the key points of nursing care during each stage.

(1) Operators' own preparation. Fully adhere to Level Ⅲ or even more strict protective measures.

(2) Patient assessment. Assess the patients' basic conditions, especially allergy history, blood glucose, coagulation function, oxygen therapy, sedation (for sober patients, pay attention to their psychological state) and catheter function status.

(3) Installation and pre-flushing. Use consumables with closed-loop management while avoiding the exposure to the patient's blood and body fluids. The corresponding instruments, pipelines and other consumables should be selected according to the planned treatment mode. All basic functions and characteristics of the consumables should be familiarized.

(4) Running. It is recommended that the initial blood draw speed is less than or equal to 35 mL/min to avoid low blood pressure which might be caused by high speed. Vital signs should be monitored as well.

(5) Parameter adjustment. When the patient's extracorporeal circulation is stable, all treatment parameters and alarm parameters should be adjusted according to the treatment mode. A sufficient amount of anticoagulant is recommended in an early stage and the anticoagulant dose should be adjusted during the maintenance period according to different treatment pressure.

(6) Weaning. Adopt "liquid gravity combined recovery method"; the recovery speed is less than or equal to 35 mL/min; after weaning, medical waste should be treated in accordance with the requirements of prevention and control for SARS-CoV-2, and the treatment room and instruments should be cleaned and disinfected as well.

(7) Recording. Make accurate records of the patients' vital signs, medication and treatment parameters for ALSS, and take notes on special conditions.

4.2 Intermittent Care

(1) Perform observation and treatment of delayed complications, such as allergic reactions, imbalance syndromes, etc.

(2) ALSS intubation care. During each shift, the medical staff should observe the patients' conditions and make records; prevent catheter-related thrombosis; carry out professional maintenance of the catheter every 48 hours.

(3) ALSS intubation and extubation care. Vascular ultrasonography should be performed before extubation. After extubation, the patient's lower limb with the intubation side should not be moved in 6 hours and the patient should lie in bed for 24 hours. After extubation, the surface of a wound should be observed.

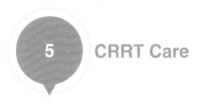

5 CRRT Care

5.1 Preparation Before Continuous Renal Replacement Treatment (CRRT)

(1) Preparation for patient. Establish effective vascular access. Generally, central vein catheterization is performed for CRRT, with the internal jugular vein preferred. A CRRT device can be integrated into the ECMO circuit if the two are applied at the same time.

(2) Prepare equipments, consumables, and ultrafiltration medication before CRRT.

5.2 In-Treatment Care

(1) Vascular access care. For patients with central venous catheterization, perform professional catheter care every 24 hours to properly fix access to avoid distortion and compression. When CRRT is integrated into ECMO treatment, the sequence and the tightness of the catheter connection should be confirmed by two nurses. Both the outflow and the inflow CRRT lines are suggested to be connected behind the oxygenator.

(2) Closely monitor consciousness and the vital signs of patients; accurately calculate the fluid inflow and outflow. Closely observe blood clotting within the cardiopulmonary bypass circuit, respond effectively to any alarms, and ensure that the machine is operating properly. Assess the electrolyte and acid-base balance in the internal environment through blood gas analysis every 4 hours. The replacement liquid should be prepared freshly and labeled clearly under strict sterile conditions.

5.3 Postoperative Care

(1) Monitor blood routine, functions of the liver and the kidney, as well as the coagulation function of the patients.

(2) Wipe the CRRT machine every 24 hours if continuous treatment is applied. Consumables and wasted liquid should be disposed in accordance with hospital requirements to avoid nosocomial infection.

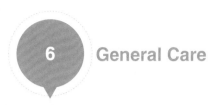

6 General Care

6.1 Monitoring

The vital signs of patients should be continuously monitored, especially changes in consciousness, respiration rate and the oxygen saturation. Observe symptoms such as cough, sputum, chest tightness, dyspnea, and cyanosis. Monitor blood gas analysis of the artery closely and timely recognize any deterioration to adjust strategies of oxygen therapy or to take urgent measures. Pay attention to ventilator associated lung injury (VALI) under high positive end-expiratory pressure (PEEP) and high-pressure support. Closely monitor changes in airway pressure, tidal volume and respiratory rate.

6.2 Aspiration Prevention

(1) Gastric retention monitor. Perform continuous post-pyloric feeding with a nutrition pump to reduce gastroesophageal reflux. Evaluate gastric motility and gastric retention with ultrasound if possible. Patients with normal gastric emptying are not recommended for routine assessment.

(2) Evaluate gastric retention every 4 hours. Re-infuse the aspirate if the gastric residual volume is less than 100 mL; otherwise, report to the attending physician.

(3) Aspiration prevention during patient transportation. Before transportation, stop nasal feeding, aspirate the gastric residues and connect the gastric tube to a negative pressure bag. During transportation, raise the patient's head up to 30°.

(4) Aspiration prevention during HFNC. Check the humidifier every

4 hours to avoid excessive or insufficient humidification. Remove any water accumulated in the tubing promptly to prevent cough and aspiration caused by the accidental entry of condensation into the airway. Keep the position of the nasal cannula higher than the machine and tubes. Promptly remove condensation in the system.

6.3 Infection Prevention

Implement strategies to prevent catheter-related bloodstream infection and catheter-related urinary tract infection.

6.4 Prevention of Skin Injuries

Prevent pressure-induced skin injuries, including device-related pressure-induced injuries, incontinence-associated dermatitis and medical adhesive-related skin injuries. Identify patients at a high risk with the Risk Assessment Scale and implement preventive strategies.

6.5 Thrombosis Prevention

Assess all patients upon admission and when their clinical conditions change with the venous thromboembolism (VTE) risk assessment model to identify those who are at a high risk and implement preventive strategies. Monitor coagulation function, D-dimer levels and VTE-related clinical manifestations.

6.6 Nutritional Support

Provide eating assistance for patients who are weak, short of breath or those with an obvious fluctuating oxygenation index. Intensify oxygenation index monitoring on such patients during meals. Provide enteral nutrition at early stages for those who are unable to eat by mouth. During each shift, adjust the enteral nutrition rate and quantity according to the tolerance of the enteral nutrition.

APPENDIX

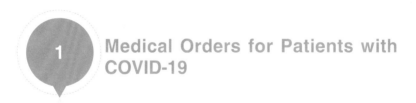

Medical Orders for Patients with COVID-19

1.1 Medical Order for Mild Patient with COVID-19

1.1.1 Treatment Order

Air isolation, blood oxygen saturation monitoring, oxygen therapy with nasal cannula.

1.1.2 Examination Order

- COVID-19 RNA Detection (Three Sites) (Sputum), qd.
- COVID-19 RNA Detection (Three Sites) (Feces), qd.
- Measurements of blood routine, biochemical profile, urine routine, stool routine + OB, coagulation function + D dimer, blood gas analysis + lactic acid, ASO + RF + CPR + CCP, ESR, PCT, ABO + RH blood type, thyroid function, cardiac enzymes + quantitative assay of serum troponin, four routine items, respiratory virus test, cytokines, G/GM test, angiotensin converting enzyme.
- Ultrasound examination of the liver, the gallbladder, the pancreas and the spleen, echocardiography and lung CT scan.

1.1.3 Medication Order

- Arbidol tablets 200 mg po tid.
- Lopinavir/ritonavir 2 tablets po q12h.
- Interferon spray 1 spray pr. nar tid.

1.2 Medical Orders for Moderate Patients with COVID-19

1.2.1 Treatment Order

Air isolation, blood oxygen saturation monitoring, oxygen therapy with nasal cannula.

1.2.2 Examination Order

- COVID-19 RNA Detection (Three Sites) (Sputum), qd.
- COVID-19 RNA Detection (Three Sites) (Feces), qd.
- Measurements of Blood routine, biochemical profile, urine routine, stool routine + OB, coagulation function + D dimer, blood gas analysis + lactic acid, ASO + RF + CPR + CCP, ESR, PCT, ABO + RH blood type, thyroid function, cardiac enzymes + quantitative assay of serum troponin, four routine items, respiratory virus test, cytokines, G/GM test, angiotensin converting enzyme
- Ultrasound examination of the liver, the gallbladder, the pancreas and the spleen, echocardiography and lung CT scan.

1.2.3 Medication Order

- Arbidol tablets 200 mg po tid.
- Lopinavir/ritonavir 2 tablets po q12h.
- Interferon spray 1 spray pr.nar tid.
- NS 100 mL + Ambroxol 30 mg ivgtt bid.

1.3 Medical Orders for Severe Patients with COVID-19

1.3.1 Treatment Order

Air isolation, blood oxygen saturation monitoring, oxygen therapy with nasal cannula.

1.3.2 Examination Order

- COVID-19 RNA Detection (Three Sites) (Sputum), qd.
- COVID-19 RNA Detection (Three Sites) (Feces), qd.

● Measurements of blood routine, biochemical profile, urine routine, stool routine + OB, coagulation function + D dimer, blood gas analysis + lactic acid, ASO + RF + CPR + CCP, ESR, PCT, ABO + RH blood type, thyroid function, cardiac enzymes + quantitative assay of serum troponin, four routine items, respiratory virus test, cytokines, G/GM test, angiotensin converting enzyme.

● Ultrasound examination of the liver, the gallbladder, the pancreas and the spleen, echocardiography and lung CT scan.

1.3.3 Medication Order

● Arbidol tablets 200 mg tid.
● Lopinavir/ritonavir 2 tablets po q12h.
● Interferon spray 1 spray pr.nar tid.
● NS 100 mL + methylprednisolone 40 mg ivgtt qd.
● NS 100 mL + pantoprazole 40 mg ivgtt qd.
● Caltrate 1 tablet qd.
● Immunoglobulin 20 g ivgtt qd.
● NS 100 mL + Ambroxol 30 mg ivgtt bid.

1.4 Medical Orders for Critical Patients with COVID-19

1.4.1 Treatment Order

Air isolation, blood oxygen saturation monitoring, oxygen therapy with nasal cannula.

1.4.2 Examination Order

● COVID-19 RNA Detection (Three Sites) (Sputum), qd
● COVID-19 RNA Detection (Three Sites) (Feces), qd
● Measurements of blood routine, ABO + RH blood type, urine routine, stool routine + OB, four routine items, respiratory virus test, thyroid function, electrocardiogram, blood gas analysis + electrolyte + lactic acid + GS, G/GM test, blood culture, ONCE.
● Measurements of blood routine, biochemical profile, coagulation

function + D dimer, blood gas analysis + lactic acid, natriuretic peptide, cardiac enzyme, quantitative assay of serum troponin, immunoglobulin + complement, cytokine, sputum culture, CRP, PCT, qd.

● Measurement of blood glucose, q6h.

● Ultrasound examination of the liver, the gallbladder, the pancreas and the spleen, echocardiography and lung CT scan.

1.4.3 Medication Order

● Arbidol tablets 200 mg po. tid.

● Lopinavir/ritonavir 2 tablets q12h (or darunavir 1 tablet qd).

● NS 10 mL + methylprednisolone 40 mg iv q12h.

● NS 100 mL + pantoprazole 40 mg ivgtt qd.

● Immunoglobulin 20 g ivgtt qd.

● Thymic peptides 1.6 mg ih biw.

● NS 10 mL + Ambroxol 30 mg iv bid.

● NS 50 mL + isoproterenol 2 mg iv-vp once.

● Human serum albumin 10 g ivgtt qd.

● NS 100 mL + piperacillin/tazobactam 4.5 g ivgtt q8h.

● Enteral nutrition suspension (Peptisorb liquid) 500 mL nasogastric feeding bid.

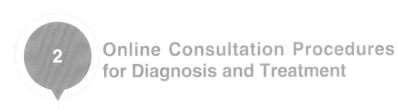

Online Consultation Procedures for Diagnosis and Treatment

2.1 Online Consultation for Diagnosis and Treatment

Instructions on FAHZU Internet+ Hospital

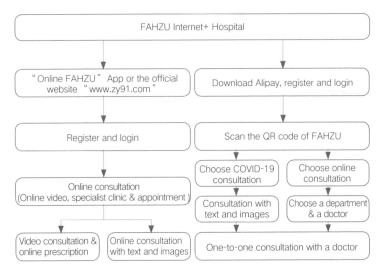

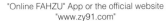

"Online FAHZU" App or the official website
"www.zy91.com"

FAHZU Internet+ Hospital
(Please scan the QR code in Alipay App.)

Please feel free to contact us.
Email: zdyy6616@126.com, zyinternational@163.com

2.2 Online Doctors' Communication Platform

Instructions on the International Medical Expert Communication Platform of The First Affiliated Hospital, Zhejiang University School of Medicine

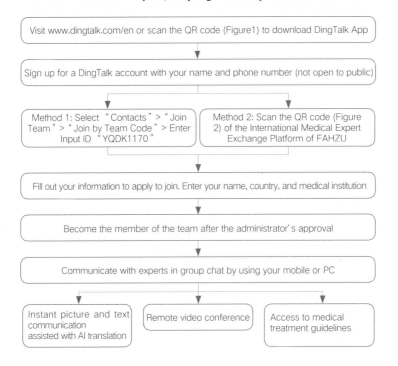

Visit www.dingtalk.com/en or scan the QR code (Figure1) to download DingTalk App

Sign up for a DingTalk account with your name and phone number (not open to public)

Method 1: Select "Contacts" > "Join Team" > "Join by Team Code" > Enter Input ID "YQDK1170"

Method 2: Scan the QR code (Figure 2) of the International Medical Expert Exchange Platform of FAHZU

Fill out your information to apply to join. Enter your name, country, and medical institution

Become the member of the team after the administrator's approval

Communicate with experts in group chat by using your mobile or PC

Instant picture and text communication assisted with AI translation

Remote video conference

Access to medical treatment guidelines

Note: Scan the QR code of Figure 3 to download user guide.

Figure1: Scan to Download DingTalk App

Figure 2: QR Code of FAHZU Communication Platform (Please scan the QR code in DingTalk App.)

Figure 3:User Guide (Please scan the QR code in DingTalk App.)

参考文献
References

[1] 国家卫生健康委，国家中医药管理局 . 新型冠状病毒肺炎诊疗方案（试行第七版）[EB/OL].(2020-03-04)[2020-03-15]. http://www.nhc.gov.cn/yzygj/s7653p/202003/46c9294a7dfe4cef80dc7f5912eb1989.shtml.

[2] 国家卫生健康委 . 新型冠状病毒肺炎防控方案（第六版）[EB/OL].(2020-03-09)[2020-03-15]. http://www.nhc.gov.cn/jkj/s3577/202003/4856d5b0458141-fa9f376853224d41d7.shtml.

[3] 中国疾病预防控制中心 . 新型冠状病毒肺炎流行病学调查指南 [EB/OL].(2020-03-09)[2020-03-15]. http://www.chinacdc.cn/jkzt/crb/zl/szkb_11803/jszl_11815/202003/t20200309_214241.html.

[4] 中国疾病预防控制中心 . 新型冠状病毒肺炎病例密切接触者调查与管理指南 [EB/OL]. (2020-03-09)[2020-03-15]. http://www.chinacdc.cn/jkzt/crb/zl/szkb_11803/jszl_11815/202003/t20200309_214241.html.

[5] 中国疾病预防控制中心 . 新型冠状病毒肺炎实验室检测技术指南 [EB/OL].(2020-03-09)[2020-03-15]. http://www.chinacdc.cn/jkzt/crb/zl/szkb_11803/jszl_11815/202003/t20200309_214241.html.

[6] 中国疾病预防控制中心 . 特定场所消毒技术指南 [EB/OL].(2020-03-09)[2020-03-15]. http://www.chinacdc.cn/jkzt/crb/zl/szkb_11803/jszl_11815/202003/t20200309_214241.html.

[7] 中国疾病预防控制中心 . 特定人群个人防护指南 [EB/OL].

(2020-03-09)[2020-03-15]. http://www.chinacdc.cn/jkzt/crb/zl/szkb_11803/jszl_11815/202003/t20200309_214241.html.

[8] 浙江省市场监督管理局 . 新冠肺炎疫情防控技术指南 第 3 部分：医疗机构：DB33/T 2241.1- 2020.

[9] 中国疾病预防控制中心 . 新型冠状病毒肺炎疫情分布 [EB/OL].[2020-03-15]. http://2019ncov.chinacdc.cn/2019-nCoV/.

[10]Wang C, Horby P W, Hayden F G, et al. A novel coronavirus outbreak of global health concern[J]. Lancet, 2020, 395(10223):470-473. DOI: 10.1016/S0140-6736(20)30185-9.

[11] 中国疾控中心在武汉华南海鲜市场检出大量新型冠状病毒 [EB/OL].(2020-01-27)[2020-03-15]. http://www.chinacdc.cn/yw_9324/202001/t20200127_211469.html.

[12] 国家卫生健康委关于新型冠状病毒肺炎暂命名事宜的通知 [EB/OL].(2020-02-07)[2020-03-15]. http://www.nhc.gov.cn/mohwsbwstjxxzx-/s2908/202002/f15dda000f6a46b2a1ea1377cd80434d.shtml.

[13]Gorbalenya A E, Baker S C, Baric R S, et al. Severe acute respiratory syndrome-related coronavirus: the species and its viruses - a statement of the Coronavirus Study Group[J/OL]. BioRxi, 2020. doi:10.1101/2020.02.07.937862.

[14]WHO. Novel Coronavirus(2019-nCoV) : situation report, 22[EB/OL].(2020-02-11) [2020-03-15]. https://www.who.int/emergencies/diseases/novel-coronavirus-2019/situation-reports/.

[15] 中华人民共和国国家卫生健康委员会疾病预防控制局 . 新型冠状病毒感染的肺炎纳入法定传染病管理 [EB/OL].(2020-01-20)[2020-03-15]. http://www.nhc.gov.cn/jkj/s7915/202001/

e4e2d5e6f01147e0a8df3f6701d49f33.shtml.

[16]Chen Y, Liang W, Yang S, et al. Human infections with the Emerging Avian Inflfluenza A H7N9 virus from wet market poultry: clinical analysis and characterisation of viral genome [J]. Lancet, 2013, 381(9881): 1916-1925. DOI: 10.1016/S0140-6736(13)60903-4.

[17]Gao H N, Lu H Z, Cao B, et al. Clinical findings in 111 cases of inflfluenza A (H7N9) virus infection[J]. N Engl J Med, 2013, 368(24): 2277-2285. DOI:10.1056/NEJMoa1305584.

[18]Liu X, Zhang Y, Xu X, et al. Evaluation of plasma exchange and continuous veno-venous hemofifiltration for the treatment of severe avian inflfluenza A (H7N9): a cohort study[J]. Ther Apher Dial, 2015, 19(2): 178-184. DOI:10.1111/1744-9987.12240.

[19] 国家感染性疾病临床医学研究中心，传染病诊治国家重点实验室. 人工肝血液净化系统应用于重型、危重型新型冠状病毒肺炎治疗的专家共识 [J]. 中华临床感染病杂志，2020, 13. DOI:10.3760/cma.j.issn.1674-2397.2020.0003.

[20]Weill D, Benden C, Corris P A, et al. A consensus document for the selection of lung transplant candidates: 2014—An update from the Pulmonary Transplantation Council of the International Society for Heart and Lung Transplantation[J]. Journal of Heart & Lung Transplantation the Offiffifficial Publication of the International Society for Heart Transplantation, 2015, 34(1): 1-15.

医嘱缩写对照表

缩写	含义
q6h	每 6 小时一次
q12h	每 12 小时一次
qd	每日一次
bid	每日两次
tid	每日三次
biw	每周两次
ONCE	临时一次
po	经口
pr.nar	鼻用
NS	生理盐水
iv	静脉内
gtt	滴注
ih	皮下注射
iv-vp	微泵静注

医院简介

浙江大学医学院附属第一医院是集医疗、教学、科研、预防、保健为一体的"国家队"医院，首批委、省共建国家医学中心、国家区域医疗中心。该医院以综合实力雄厚、医疗质量过硬、学科特色鲜明享誉海内外。医院综合排名全国第14位，连续10年保持浙江第1位，其中传染病学连续6年蝉联全国第1位。

浙江大学医学院附属第一医院建院于1947年，是浙江大学创建的首家附属医院。医院拥有庆春、余杭、之江等六大院区，床位数4000余张，2019年门（急）诊量达500万人次，出院21.43万人次。医院现有职工6500余人，正高职称364人，副高职称545人，拥有多位中国工程院院士、国家杰出青年科学基金获得者、"长江学者"特聘教授等顶尖人才。

医院承担了多项国家科技重大专项、国家重点研发计划、国家自然科学基金等国家级课题，近10年每年到位科研经费保持在1亿元以上，其中有6年超过2亿元。多年来，医院在器官移植、胰腺疾病、传染病、血液病、肾脏病、泌尿系疾病、临床药学等学科领域享有盛名，建立了现代化胰腺癌规范诊治创新技术体系，成功开展肝脏、胰腺、肺、肾、小肠和心脏等多器官移植手术。自2003年以来，医院在抗击SARS、H7N9和COVID-19过程中积累了丰富的经验，先后在 New England Journal of Medicine、The Lancet、Nature、Science 等主刊上发表学术论文多篇，取得授权专利300余项，出版专著200余部。

　　长期以来，医院持续推动全球范围内的交流合作，与美国斯坦福大学、约翰·霍普金斯医院等 30 余家世界顶尖高校和医疗机构建立了深厚的合作关系。此外，医院将先进技术和优秀人才向匈牙利、印度尼西亚、马来西亚等中东欧和东南亚国家辐射，取得了丰硕的医学外交成果。

　　医院牢记"以卓越的医疗品质促进人类健康"的使命，坚持"科技引领，创新发展，科学管理，优质服务"的发展思路，秉承"严谨求实"的核心价值观，致力于为患者提供高品质的医疗服务，争取早日成为国际一流的医学中心。

Overview of FAHZU

The First Affiliated Hospital, Zhejiang University School of Medicine (FAHZU) has evolved into a national-level hospital integrating health care, medical education, scientific research and preventative care. It is also one of the first National Medical Science Centers and National-level Regional Medical Centers co-built by the National Health Commission and provincial government. It boasts strong overall strength, high medical quality and distinctive disciplinary features both at home and abroad. It ranked 14th in terms of overall strength, continuing to be the provincial best for 10 consecutive years, and Infectious Diseases continued to be the national best for 6 consecutive years.

Founded in 1947, FAHZU is the earliest affiliated hospital of Zhejiang University. With 6 campuses (Qingchun, Yuhang, Zhijiang, etc.), it has over 4000 beds. The year 2019 has seen 5 million outpatients and emergency visits and 214,300 discharges. There are more than 6500 employees including many members of the Chinese Academy of Engineering, National Distinguished Young Scholars, and Changjiang Distinguished Professors.

FAHZU has been devoted to many national research projects including National Science and Technology Major Projects, National Key R&D Programs and National Natural Science Foundation Programs. The annual funding for scientific research has reached 100 million RMB for 10 consecutive years. In the past 6 years it has exceeded 200 million RMB. Over the years, it has successfully developed a number of renowned programs including organ transplantation, pancreatic diseases, infectious diseases, hematology, nephrology, urology, clinical pharmacy, etc., and set up a modernized and innovative approach to the standardized diagnosis and treatment of pancreatic cancer. It is also an integrated provider of liver, pancreas, lung, kidney, intestine and heart transplantation. In the fights against SARS, H7N9 avian flu and COVID-19, it has gained rich experience and fruitful outcomes.

As a result, its medical professionals have published many articles in journals such as *New England Journal of Medicine*, *The Lancet*, *Nature* and *Science*. More than 300 patents have been granted and nearly 200 monographs have been published.

FAHZU has been extensively engaged into overseas exchanges and collaboration. It has established partnerships with over 30 prestigious universities and medical institutions around the world including Stanford University, Johns Hopkins Hospital, etc. Productive achievements have also been accomplished through exchange of our medical experts and technologies with Hungary, Indonesia, Malaysia and other Central and Eastern European and Southeastern Asian countries.

Shouldering the mission of promoting human health by outstanding medical care services, FAHZU adheres to the guidelines of innovative development, sound management, and optimum medical services, and to the core value of seeking truth with prudence. It has devoted itself to providing high-quality medical care to patients, striving to become world-class medical center.

图书在版编目（CIP）数据

新型冠状病毒肺炎临床救治手册：浙大一院临床实践经验 / 梁廷波主编. -- 杭州：浙江大学出版社，2020.4

ISBN 978-7-308-20117-9

Ⅰ. ①新… Ⅱ. ①梁… Ⅲ. ①日冕形病毒－病毒病－肺炎－诊疗－手册 Ⅳ. ①R563.1-62

中国版本图书馆CIP数据核字(2020)第053425号

新型冠状病毒肺炎临床救治手册：浙大一院临床实践经验

梁廷波　主编

责任编辑	张　鸽　张凌静　冯其华　殷晓彤
责任校对	冯其华
美术编辑	续设计
出版发行	浙江大学出版社
	（杭州市天目山路148号　邮政编码　310007）
	（网址：http://www.zjupress.com）
排　　版	杭州林智广告有限公司
印　　刷	浙江省邮电印刷股份有限公司
开　　本	889mm×1194mm　1/32
印　　张	6.5
字　　数	166千
版 印 次	2020年4月第1版　2020年4月第1次印刷
书　　号	ISBN 978-7-308-20117-9
定　　价	68.00元
